Living Well with Kidney Failure

Living Well with Kidney Failure

A guide to living with kidney failure

Juliet Auer
Dip. Professional Social Work,
CQSW, M.Phil (Research)
Renal Patient Support Manager, Oxford Kidney Unit

CLASS PUBLISHING • LONDON

Text © Juliet Auer 2005
Typography © Class Publishing (London) Ltd 2005

Printing history
First published 2005

The author and publisher welcome feedback from the users of this book.
Please contact the publishers.

Class Publishing (London) Ltd, Barb House, Barb Mews, London W6 7PA
Telephone: 020 7371 2119
Fax: 020 7371 2878 [International +4420]
Email: post@class.co.uk

The information presented in this book is accurate and current to the best of the author's knowledge. The author and publisher, however, make no guarantee as to, and assume no responsibility for, the correctness, sufficiency or completeness of such information or recommendation. The reader is advised to consult a doctor regarding all aspects of individual health care.

A CIP catalogue record for this book is available from the British Library

ISBN 1 85959 112 4

Edited by Richenda Milton-Thompson

Indexed by Valerie Elliston

Line drawings by David Woodroffe

Typeset by Martin Bristow

Printed and bound in Finland by WS Bookwell, Juva

Contents

Foreword

Chronic renal failure lasts a lifetime – intruding on every part of life. It is hard to imagine how daunting it must be to fact the diagnosis and all its implications for the first time. This cheerful book will be a great help and encouragement to patients and their families trying to become experts on renal failure. The technical aspects of dialysis and transplantation are here, but the really valuable core is the explanation of the day-to-day issues like relationships, holidays, work and leisure.

Juliet Auer has a deep understanding of the many ways that renal failure affects the lives of patients, having spent more than twenty years listening and talking (in that order!) to them. This book distils her wisdom and experience but charmingly she has let the patients speak for themselves. Doctors and nurses will find this a humbling read, which will increase their admiration for the courage of many of their patients. Patients and their families should be reassured by it, learning that they are not the first to feel the way they do, and that support and understanding are at hand.

C G Winearls

Christopher G Winearls D.Phil, FRCP London
Clinical Director, Oxford Kidney Unit

Introduction

Having worked with kidney patients for over 25 years, I have seen many changes and improvements in treatment. However, this book is not a comprehensive guide to the medical and nursing aspects of illness and treatment. These are mentioned briefly where it is necessary to explain the effects of the illness and treatment on daily life.

This book is about living with kidney failure. It celebrates the fullness of life which kidney patients can attain. It is based on the experiences of a number of very different people for whom kidney failure has become part of an otherwise full and rewarding life.

Most of the contributors are on the waiting list for a kidney transplant; a few are not, either due to their own choice, or because their medical condition makes them unsuitable for major surgery. Four have now had transplants, so are able to talk about living well in this situation too.

Naturally, people who make a success of their life after a diagnosis of kidney failure will, from time to time, have setbacks or bad patches. In any chronic, life-long condition lasting over a period of several decades, it would be unrealistic to pretend that life can be trouble-free all the time. Many of them, however, continue to *live* with their kidney failure and, more importantly, to live with it *well*.

After talking at length with the contributors, I was filled with admiration for their courage and determination. This was a different sort of courage from that sometimes shown in an emergency – great heroism in the short term. But arguably, people who are living with kidney failure are achieving something more difficult and more admirable. Dealing successfully with a life-long condition requires, more than anything, perseverance. This quality, and many others too, are evident in the stories they share with us throughout this book. These stories will be an inspiration to others facing a diagnosis of kidney failure and the need for treatment.

Dialysis in the beginning

Before the 1960s, chronic kidney failure was a death sentence. During the 1960s, regular dialysis became a possibility, but dialysis in hospital was limited. Very few units provided it, and dialysis machines were expensive and far between. These scarce facilities were used to train the most capable patients, usually young working people with families to support, so that they might dialyse themselves at home. Treatment took up to ten hours a session, and setting up the cumbersome machines for each dialysis, which involved cleaning and re-using all the equipment, could take additional hours. In those days, dialysis was quite an ordeal.

Once regular dialysis was established, it became evident that there were also long-term complications of kidney failure which were not helped by dialysis treatment. These included anaemia (lack of red blood cells) and weakening of the bones. At the time, these problems were poorly understood and hard to treat. Patients needed regular blood transfusions to combat the anaemia. There were also complications caused by the treatment itself. Patients developed inflammation of the joints, especially in the shoulders and wrists, due to the body's reaction against the artificial membranes used in the dialysis machines. A further problem soon became apparent, when some patients developed a type of dementia found to be caused by aluminium, absorbed either from the water used in dialysis or from medication. This became known as 'dialysis dementia'.

Kidney failure was no longer a death sentence, but in some ways it had become a *life* sentence. Quality of life for those early patients was severely limited and a transplant was the only hope of leading a full life. It is no wonder that kidney failure and dialysis were dreaded, and that the media painted a gloomy picture which still colours the public perception of the treatment.

Progress, since then, has been dramatic. Dialysis is now available to anybody who needs it and wants it, regardless of age or other medical conditions. There is a choice of treatment between haemodialysis (the kidney machine, see page 33) and peritoneal dialysis (see page 36). Haemodialysis now takes, on average, only three or four hours per session, and the preparation is relatively quick and straightforward these days. Treatment is performed either at home or in hospital, two or three times a week, and most units can arrange evening dialysis if you want to work full time. Peritoneal dialysis is home-based, and can either be done during the day, or overnight (see page 37). In the early days of continuous ambulatory peritoneal dialysis (CAPD), patients carried the empty plastic bag in their pocket or taped to their abdomen, after draining the fluid in. Now, this bag is disconnected, making the treatment more acceptable from the aesthetic point of view.

The complications of kidney failure have been greatly reduced due to:

• Early treatment to prevent the development of bone problems;

- The discovery and manufacture of a hormone called erythropoietin (see page 27), which is able to correct anaemia caused by kidney failure;

- The development of dialysis membranes which are 'bio-compatible', kinder to your body, and do not cause inflammatory deposits in the joints;

- Improved water treatment, which has eliminated the problem of 'dialysis dementia'(see page 2);

- Bicarbonate dialysis, which is a far gentler treatment than treatment with the original dialysis fluids;

- Better PD solutions, which are likely to be more compatible with your body tissue, so less damaging to the peritoneal membrane;

- Advances in PD systems which have reduced the likelihood of infections, previously a major problem for PD patients.

With these advances in treatment, patients need not be afraid of dialysis in the way they used to be. As one patient's wife said: 'Contrary to what is reported in the popular press, it is not transplants that save lives when kidneys fail, it is dialysis'. Dialysis can now be a viable long-term alternative to transplantation, giving patients a good quality of life. Life no longer needs to be 'put on hold' until a donor kidney becomes available – indeed some patients now make a positive choice to remain on dialysis rather than receive a transplant.

The differences between patients

During my time working with kidney patients, the single most interesting (and puzzling) thing, has been the difference in people's reactions. Some seem to cope well and make the most of life, and others let the illness and treatment 'win', and rule their lives. The latter group seem to have neither time nor enthusiasm left for maintaining previous ambitions, pastimes and pleasures. They seem resigned to becoming invalids. 'Life' has become 'kidney failure', and it is a full-time occupation. They are not happy people.

Those who have made the most of their situation, however, seem to have relegated their kidney failure to the position it deserves. They regard it as a means to an end, no more to be neglected than other life-sustaining functions, but belonging in the background rather than at the centre of their lives.

It is not easy to be a dialysis patient (any more than living with the side effects of transplant surgery is always easy). Nor are 'successful' patients always cheerful and problem free. However, there are 168 hours in each week. Dialysis treatment takes about 15–20 hours a week, we sleep for perhaps a further 56 hours a week, leaving 92 hours a week in which to make the most of life without thinking about dialysis at all. In addition, many of those who are coping well use their treatment time to work, read, surf the Internet or write letters, so that even less time is lost to dialysis.

It might be tempting to think that those who 'do well' are probably those lucky ones who feel well on dialysis, and have no complications or additional illnesses. If they are medically fitter, surely they will be better able to lead a normal life. While this is true in some cases, there are plenty of others who do not fit into this pattern. For example, there are some patients with many problems additional to kidney failure, such as diabetes, heart conditions and even cancers, who nevertheless continue to lead active and rewarding lives.

A shining example of this was a man I met two years ago, who has recently died. He was in his fifties and had kidney failure caused by myeloma, a cancer of the bone marrow. He was told from the outset that his condition was incurable, but with chemotherapy and dialysis he might live some years. He had recently taken time off work, because he felt very ill as his kidneys declined, but the moment he started dialysis, he returned to part-time work in a supermarket warehouse, fitting it round his chemotherapy and kidney treatment. At weekends he took his wife on short breaks to the Isle of Wight where they had friends. He had two dogs which he took for long walks. He was always cheerful, always friendly and concerned for others, and always positive. When his first chemotherapy course finished, he thought he should work longer hours, so went in to work after his morning dialysis as well as on the days in between. His myeloma had responded to the first chemotherapy course, but, six months later, failed to respond to the second course. He did not even cut his hours of work, in spite of getting weaker and more tired. He now needed regular blood transfusions. In fact he worked until a fortnight before his death from myeloma.

But there are other kidney patients who, with no other problems, seem to give up and become all too ready to see themselves as invalids.

I felt that finding out what contributed to these differences might help new (and maybe established) patients to create a better quality of life. Were there any common factors shared by these 'successful', optimistic patients? Was it, perhaps, a question of age, sex, occupation, treatment type, financial position? Could it be that there was a single 'successful' personality type?

However, having talked to many patients with kidney failure, there seem to be no reliable pointers to help predict which patients will cope well with their new situation. This category covers both sexes, and encompasses a whole range of ages, ethnic backgrounds, occupations and financial situations. The 'successful' copers also appear to have widely differing personalities and ways of dealing with their situation. There seem to be as many ways of being a 'patient who copes successfully' as there are patients themselves.

It is important to hear what patients themselves say, since they are the experts – the only ones who know what it is really like to depend on dialysis to stay alive, and yet to create a rewarding way of life. It is they who, more than anyone, can give us pointers towards successful adaptation. The contributors to this book are not 'exceptional', at least not in the sense of running marathons, cycling from Land's End to John O'Groats or climbing mountains – things that some rare kidney patients have achieved, but that most 'ordinary' people could never aspire to. They are like you and me. We will meet many of them in this book.

Introducing the contributors

The table below presents brief details about contributors, in a convenient form, for you to refer to. For reasons of confidentiality, names have been changed but contributors' own words are used throughout the text.

Name	Occupation	Treatment
Andrew aged 44	Builder	On evening hospital haemodialysis
Chris aged 29	Gardener	On evening hospital haemodialysis
Frances aged 69	Supermarket checkout worker	On continuous ambulatory peritoneal dialysis (CAPD)
George aged 35	Self employed in IT	On evening hospital haemodialysis

Name	Occupation	Treatment
Helen aged 35	Works in a supermarket	Haemodialysis, now transplanted for 8 years
Indira aged 48	Social Worker	On automated peritoneal dialysis, followed by transplant
Jenny aged 56	Housewife and artist	On home haemodialysis
Joyce aged 70	Carer	Husband on hospital haemodialysis
Laura aged 45	Aromatherapist	On automated peritoneal dialysis
Keith aged 44	Community Education Officer – Fire Service	Haemodialysis, hospital and home, CAPD, now transplanted for 17 years
Mary aged 71	Retired midwife	On hospital haemodialysis
Paul aged 36	Unemployed chef/ voluntary worker	On hospital haemodialysis
Reg aged 77	Retired bricklayer	On hospital haemodialysis
Rhys aged 49	Deputy headmaster	On automated peritoneal dialysis
Robert aged 50	Project manager	On evening hospital haemodialysis, followed by transplant

1
Diagnosis

If you have just been told that your kidneys are failing, you probably feel very shocked, frightened and alone. Your life has suddenly changed and the future is full of uncertainty. This is how the diagnosis affected the people who are contributing to this book.

Although they are all, now, leading full lives, it was not always so for any of them. They all needed time to come to terms with kidney failure and had setbacks and low patches. Many, like Chris, said that the diagnosis was one of the worst times.

I remember it so clearly. The consultant said to me 'Do you want the good news or the bad news? The good news is that we have caught you in time, the bad news is that your kidneys are going to pack up completely in the next two weeks'. I only heard that I had two weeks to live. My mind was racing, and I wasn't really listening after that. I was thinking how to break the news to my family, and how to plan my funeral. But all I said was 'You must have got the wrong patient – that's not me', and I walked towards the door, and fainted!

Chris

This was the reaction of a young man who felt reasonably well and had no idea that he had reached 'end-stage renal failure' (the term for kidney failure severe enough to need dialysis). It may be extreme, but it demonstrates several points that can be common to people receiving bad news.

- **The first is that he recollected the event in painful detail,** just as most people can recall the exact circumstances when they heard about the shooting of President Kennedy, the death of Princess Diana, or the attack on the World Trade Centre. The strong feelings we experience seem to etch the moment on our minds.

- **The second is that, at the time, his mind completely ignored the 'good news'** and heard only the bad. After grabbing the bad news, he stopped listening and tried to work out the implications of the fact that he was going to die. Under extreme stress, we are unable to hear or think clearly. We often focus only on the worst thing that has been said.

- **The third is Chris's next response – disbelief.** Part of his mind found the news so unbearable that he rejected it completely, and said that the doctor had got the wrong patient.

- **Finally, he tried to escape, to run away**, by leaving the room. But the shock and adrenaline-rush may have upset his blood pressure, so that the act of getting up to leave caused him to pass out.

Chris was diagnosed very late, so had no time to get used to the fact that his kidneys were not working as well as they should. Had he had time to face the situation gradually, taking in a little at a time, he would certainly have found the news less traumatic.

Rhys had a little more time, about five months from diagnosis to dialysis, but his reactions again show how the mind shrinks from accepting the situation:

> *I went to the GP because I was having to get up to pass urine frequently at night. I immediately felt that something was badly wrong, because the timescale from getting the blood test to being referred to the kidney specialist ('just to make sure' as the doctor put it; 'sure of what?' I wondered) was only a week. Given the pressures on the NHS this made me very suspicious! I found myself sitting in the waiting room among all the other renal patients, and everything inside me was screaming 'you're in the wrong place'. I thought he would give me a check-up, throw a few pills at me and I would be on my way. The doctor had to be very firm with me to get me to accept the severity of the situation. I always remember he said 'Please understand, you are very ill', and I said 'But I don't do 'sick'!*

> *Rhys*

Rhys's mind (like Chris's) was operating on two levels at once. He suspected the worst, and was acutely sensitive to the fact that his GP was worried and that his appointment was arranged too quickly to be routine, yet he reacted with disbelief – 'incredulity' is his word – when told his condition was indeed serious. His reaction was, 'I thought those things happened to other people'.

Here again, in spite of denying that anything serious could be wrong,

Rhys reports that his mind was racing to cope with the implications of the news:

After seeing the kidney doctor, I had to have blood taken, which was bad because I'm needle-phobic, and the nurses were saying to me that I would have to stop work and prepare for kidney treatment. It all sounded very gloomy. My daughter was just going to college and I'd only just taken out a new mortgage, so my mind was racing about how I would cope with everything financially, if I had to stop work.

Rhys

Chris and Rhys were both referred rapidly to a kidney doctor once they had visited their GPs, but this does not always happen. The following situation is, luckily, fairly rare:

I had been ill for over six months – constant sickness, severe headaches, and my GP said 'You are depressed, you need antidepressants'. It was during the summer, and I usually get hay fever. I was breathless and wheezy, so he gave me stronger tablets for hay fever. I went for eye tests to see if that was the cause of the headaches, but everyone was telling me there was nothing wrong. One day I was so ill that I had to be admitted to hospital. I was admitted in the morning, and in the afternoon they told me 'Your kidneys have failed'. I said 'How can you say that? I worked all yesterday. I know I have been unwell, but it can't be as bad as that!' And they said, 'this is why you have been unwell'. I was just so angry, *so confused and angry. And there was disbelief, I said 'I am still at work – surely you mean my kidneys are failing' and they said 'No, they* have failed.'

Indira

Indira has admitted to two further feelings commonly experienced at some stage during the early weeks of coming to terms with the diagnosis – *confusion* and *anger*. Another common reaction is to blame the injustice of fate – to say 'What have I done to deserve this? I have always tried to be a good and kind person', and to be angry with the unfairness of life. In her case, the anger was directed mostly at the professionals who had not recognised the symptoms produced by her failing kidneys at an earlier stage. (Unfortunately, doctors are human, and they can make mistakes.)

Many people feel that earlier diagnosis could have prevented the need for dialysis. In some cases this may be true. In most cases, however, earlier diagnosis might have delayed the need for dialysis treatment for some months or even a year, but would not have prevented the kidneys from failing at a later stage.

When they told me, my first reaction was 'Why me? What have I done? I haven't led a mad lifestyle, I'm not an alcoholic'. And the thing that annoyed me more than anything was that they couldn't find out why it had happened.

Frances

Another reaction that is quite common is described by Frances. Many people feel that they may have caused the problem themselves. Kidney failure is hardly ever someone's fault. Drinking too much alcohol may damage the liver, heart and brain – but not the kidneys. Smoking seriously damages the lungs and heart, and can clog up your blood vessels. But it is seldom the *main* reason for kidney failure.

It is not at all uncommon for doctors to be unable to say why the kidneys have failed. If they are already small and scarred, there is nothing that can be done to help them, so there is no point in searching for a reason. If the failing kidneys are still normal in size, it is worth finding out the cause, because medication may help to delay or prevent further damage. In such cases, a biopsy may be done. This involves taking a small piece of kidney tissue and examining it under a microscope. If this shows that there is inflammation (e.g. from glomerulonephritis, see page 11), steroids may be prescribed to slow down the damage.

One of the most important benefits of early diagnosis is that the patient has time to come to terms with what is happening, to adapt to the future need for treatment, and avoid the extreme shock that several of our first contributors experienced. It also allows the kidney unit team to prepare you, physically and mentally, so that you will be as fit as possible when the date for starting dialysis approaches. Alternatively, there may be time to assess your fitness for a kidney transplant. Some people go on the waiting list, and receive a kidney from somebody who has died, before the need for dialysis treatment. If you have a family member or close friend who wishes to donate a kidney to you (see page 54) the operation can be planned so that you receive a so-called 'living donor transplant' before you need dialysis.

In Frances's case, early diagnosis gave her time to adjust to the fact that she would eventually need treatment, but she still resisted starting dialysis:

I wasn't a very easy patient – not at first. When the consultant told me that my kidneys were going to fail, I just wouldn't believe it. I said to him,

'I feel well and I just cannot accept it' – and I wouldn't! It took a long time for me to accept it. I started off going to clinic once every three months, then once every two months, then once every month. In all, it was another two years before I needed to start treatment. Things were slowly getting worse, and I think I knew something was wrong, because my skin was getting terrible – dry and scaly and the itching was unbearable. I would be in tears with it.

And finally I had a routine blood test at my GP's. He rang on a Friday evening and said 'I think you should go to the Kidney Unit immediately, I have rung them to let them know'. And I said, 'No, I feel fine, I'll wait till Monday'. I told my husband about it then went to have a bath. When I came down he said 'You are going in tomorrow. The kidney unit rang and said that if you don't, you'll be coming in with a flashing blue light'. So that was it!

Frances

Whether people are diagnosed early or late, they go through similar psychological reactions. But those who are diagnosed early have time to work through their shock, anger and disbelief. Even so, Frances found it hard to accept that the time had finally arrived when she should start dialysis.

Whether the diagnosis is early or late depends partly on the cause of the kidney failure. In around 30 per cent of cases, the cause of a person's kidney failure is unknown. Many of the patients in this group have kidneys that are smaller than average, but this is not always the case. For the remaining 70 per cent of patients, there are six fairly common causes and a large number of rare ones. The common causes are:

- **Diabetes** – this is not primarily a disease of the kidneys, but it causes damage to all the small blood vessels in the body, including those in the kidneys and at the back of the eyes, which can cause blindness. Long-term damage to the small blood vessels in the kidneys can cause kidney failure. Diabetes is the most common known cause of kidney failure, and affects up to 20 per cent of patients.

- **Glomerulonephritis** – where the tiny filtering units inside the kidney become inflamed, eventually causing scarring, and shrinkage of the kidney. This is usually caused by the body's own defence system turning against the kidneys and attacking healthy tissue. (There are other illnesses caused by a similar mistaken reaction on the part of the body, for example rheumatoid arthritis, where the body attacks the lining of the joints, causing swelling and damage.)

- **Pyelonephritis** – a condition that may start in early childhood. In some cases, repeated kidney infections gradually damage the kidneys, again causing scarring and shrinkage.

- **Polycystic kidney disease** – this is the only common cause that can be inherited from parents and passed on to children. Cysts form on the kidneys, and may become very large. Over a long period, these cysts replace healthy kidney tissue, until there is not enough of it left to function properly. These cysts are not malignant (cancerous) swellings, but usually cause the kidneys to become several times their normal size.

- **Obstruction** – if there is a blockage somewhere in the kidneys or in the tubes leading to the bladder (ureters), or in the bladder outflow tube (urethra), the kidneys may become damaged by the pressure of urine unable to pass normally. Blockages can be caused by kidney or bladder stones, but the most common cause is enlargement of the prostate gland (in older men).

- **Problems in the blood supply to the kidneys** – as one gets older, various blood vessels in the body may become furred-up or narrowed. The kidneys need a rich blood supply to work well, and if this supply is reduced by narrow blood vessels (renal artery stenosis) they become damaged. Patients with narrowed blood vessels usually have an increase in their blood pressure (hypertension) which is also a cause of kidney damage. This is a common cause in older people, and there does appear to be a relationship with smoking while young.

People with diabetes and those with polycystic kidneys, are usually aware that there may be a problem with their kidney function in the future. Those attending a diabetic clinic will be monitored for changes both in the eyes and the kidneys. Those who know that family members had polycystic kidneys, may get advance warning from screening and checks on their blood pressure. High blood pressure can be a symptom of polycystic kidney disease.

Our next two contributors, Mary and Andrew, both have polycystic kidney disease. Both knew well in advance that there could be problems – yet both found it hard to accept kidney failure when it happened.

I knew that I might have polycystic kidneys, because my father and uncle died of kidney failure from adult polycystic kidney disease when they were in their fifties. It was confirmed that I had it too when I was pregnant with my daughter, but it didn't cause me much trouble. I went for check-ups for the next 30 years, and I thought I had escaped, because I got to 63 and still didn't need dialysis.

It was a great shock when they told me I would soon need treatment. In the next couple of years, I kept going because I loved my work – I was a community midwife. My consultant kept saying that I should take things a bit easier, but I was determined to prove I could do it! I worked to 65 and I have to admit it was getting harder and harder, but I didn't want to give in.

I dreaded going on dialysis and put it off and put it off, until I felt really ill. I should have started earlier, because I felt so much better when I went on treatment.

Mary

Mary had convinced herself that she would never need dialysis; In her family, those with polycystic kidney disease had reached that point far earlier, so she believed that she was in the clear. Andrew had a different view:

I had a pretty good idea at a very early age that I might have a problem with my kidneys. Nine years ago I had a scan, because I passed some blood in my urine. That showed that I had lost 60 per cent of my kidneys. I was attending renal clinic for two or three years before I needed dialysis. My mind set has always been that 'I am not a kidney patient', so I tried to carry on as normal. I go on how I feel, and I ignore everything else – what the blood tests show and that sort of thing. That's how I cope. I suppose I am 'in denial'.

Andrew

Andrew accepted that he needed treatment with one part of his mind, but has completely rejected the diagnosis in another part and tells himself, he is 'not a kidney patient'. As he himself says, he is using a technique called 'denial', which can be a useful way of coping with things that we do not want to accept, but which does have some dangers if carried to extremes (see page 114).

When Robert was told that he had kidney failure and would need dialysis within a couple of years, his reaction was similar:

I didn't believe it because I was healthy, I was normal, I was working and

everything was fine. Now I'm on dialysis, I still don't believe it to a degree –
I still don't believe it's me this is happening to.

Robert

Although treatment for kidney failure has changed and improved over the years, the feelings that people experience when confronted with bad news, have not changed at all. This is the way that Jenny describes her reactions, when she faced the need for dialysis nearly a quarter of a century ago:

I remember the diagnosis vividly, although it was 24 years ago. Attitudes of medical staff – the way things are handled, have changed dramatically since then. In those days you just accepted what you were told, and shut up and got on with it. I was in complete denial. They were saying 'It's this bad' but I said 'no it's not, there's been a mistake'. I did feel ill, but I thought 'It will go away. I haven't got time for this at the moment. I am 31 years old and have two young children'.

It was about eleven months before I actually needed dialysis. I kept putting it off – I wouldn't give in. I told myself everything was fine, but in fact I would get up in the morning, take the children to school, get the supper ready when I got back home and then go to bed until late afternoon. I was so tired and breathless I could hardly drag myself upstairs. I would pick the children up from school, manage to stay up with them until about 7.00 pm and then I went back to bed – and that seemed to me a better way of life than dialysing!

My husband was so supportive, but if he said 'Come along love, you ought to start dialysing', I would throw a wobbly and start crying and say 'You're not going to have to do this, it's me, and it's for life!'

Jenny

So far, we have heard a number of rather similar stories from people about the negative side of the diagnosis. Although people describe themselves as 'stunned' or 'shocked', unable to believe or accept the situation, these feelings can themselves be a protection against receiving bad news. Denial and disbelief enable us to cope with the early stages of adjustment. This allows us to accept things bit by bit when we are ready to do so. There were, in fact, some positive aspects mentioned by some of the people who told their stories. Like Rhys, for example:

In some respects it was a relief, because I had been thinking I was a wimp. I had terrible lethargy and was falling asleep in the afternoon. I was struggling to keep going. I thought I just needed to get out there and exercise, because I had become unfit. The kidney failure was an explanation.

Rhys

Others have told me that they were desperately worried by their weight loss and lack of energy, privately believing that they were suffering from the late stages of cancer. This is very understandable, since kidney failure makes one feel generally unwell, with poor appetite and, in the later stages, vomiting. Naturally there is weight loss, which can be a symptom of other illnesses too. These people confessed they were relieved to hear that their problem was kidney failure, since they knew that they could be successfully treated.

Where does negativity start?

Sadly, a new patient is unlikely to hear much of the 'good news' when attending hospital. Their first experience of kidney failure is usually in an outpatient clinic. Patients often talk to each other in clinic, because waiting is inevitable. Unfortunately, as in the newspapers, it tends to be the bad news that is reported and discussed. Every waiting room has its horror stories and complainers. Often the chief topics of conversation are the transport mix-ups, the cancelled appointments, the postponed operations, the procedures that were uncomfortable and the dietary restrictions. While it can be comforting to know that one is not the only person to have this sort of tiresome experience, it can also be alarming as each story tries to top the previous one. I have watched new patients, silent, but with ears pricked like startled hares, absorbing the 'bad news'. Finally, they get in to see the doctor, and are told, in all probability, that things are under control and going well. 'Ah' they think, 'I know what it's really going to be like because I have heard it from the people who know!'.

How many outpatients tell their neighbours when everything goes according to plan, or painlessly, or on time? How many talk about their interests and enthusiasms away from the hospital, or mention that they are going back to work when their appointment is over? Those who are 'quietly getting on with their lives' are, indeed, doing so *quietly*. As a result, the new patient gets a distorted view of what is in store and seldom hears a positive view of the future.

Matters may become even worse when a patient is admitted to have dialysis access (see pages 33–7) created. The ward (usually 20–30 beds for a unit covering a thousand patients with kidney failure) is mostly occupied by people who are very sick. Due to the need for dialysis to be readily available, some patients may be on the kidney ward for reasons only indirectly connected with kidney failure. Some will be very elderly and frail, some will have had amputations due to diabetic or circulation problems, some may have had heart attacks or strokes. But they are all there on the renal ward. 'So this is what will happen to me', thinks the new patient, unaware of the silent majority out there at home, or at work, or at play.

In this book we will hear from some of the people who make up this silent majority.

2
Preparing for dialysis

Our contributors produced a variety of feelings and reactions to the days and months following their diagnosis. They also expressed very different views on the information they were given to help them prepare for treatment.

> *I saw the consultant a week after the diagnosis and asked him questions about work, lifestyle and so on, and he said, 'I have known people who have worked 60 hours a week while on dialysis – so what's the problem?' And I thought 'If other people have done it, so can I' He had worked out what sort of person I am. He saw how I ticked and he gave me the information in the best possible way for me.*
>
> **Rhys**

> *My consultant talked me through all the procedures, but it was just in one ear and out the other. I wasn't ready to hear anything. The trouble was, that when I calmed down enough to listen, I didn't get nearly enough information. There was no pre-dialysis education at my first hospital, so I had to go on the Internet to find things out.*
>
> **Chris**

> *I was diagnosed too late to attend any information meeting. They gave me a book but you don't read it properly straight away, you can't really concentrate. I skipped through it each time, and the nurse kept saying 'Haven't you read the book yet?'*
>
> **Indira**

These three people were all diagnosed too late to receive the preparation that would have helped them adjust to their situation. Robert and Andrew were luckier, but while Robert was eager to know more about what lay ahead, and benefited from information, Andrew was unwilling to face things.

I was invited to a seminar on different types of dialysis, and another on transplant, and talked to people who were on treatment. I had the right information at the right time.

Robert

I don't think you can be given enough information. Everyone is so different. They tell you what you can expect, and the first time that doesn't happen, you think 'Do they know what they're talking about?' I went to the pre-dialysis and transplant seminars, though I didn't want to go to them and I didn't take much on board from them. I took all the information home with me, and said 'I'll worry about all that when I'm nearer needing dialysis'.

Andrew

Although preparation through group seminars is useful, people are all different, so general information cannot cover everybody's needs. Rhys points out that too much information at one time may be hard to take in. Indira stresses the needs of those who may not speak or read English, and therefore need information in their own language, or from visual material like videos.

There's only a certain amount of information you can take in at a time – especially when you have been stunned by the diagnosis. Your brain is fully occupied trying to come to terms with that. I was given a book about kidney failure, which my wife read to me, because I didn't feel I could tackle it at that point.

Rhys

A lot of Asian women don't speak English and may not understand the information they are given. I think there should be videos to show them about the different treatments. Patients need information directly, not through an interpreter, and not through the family. In my work I sometimes have to use an interpreter for clients, and I know enough about the Indian languages to say that the information was not being given fully. If you don't have the information, you cannot be in control of what is happening, and to be in control is very important. Asian women may not seem to 'take charge', but especially in the home, they are very much in charge.

Indira

Preparation for dialysis falls into two very different categories – practical and psychological. You and your kidney unit need to address both of these areas if you are to be well prepared for dialysis. There may be several years available for this process, or the whole thing may need to be achieved in a week. Six months to a year is probably about the ideal length of time in which to complete the preparation, but this will not be possible if the diagnosis is late. If it is longer, people can convince themselves that it will never happen, and then the whole initial process of acceptance has to be worked-through again. If shorter, it may be difficult to plan any changes that would make dialysis go more smoothly, such as negotiating with employers or setting up child care.

Pre-dialysis seminars

I'd had seven or eight years knowing my kidneys would fail one day, and all that time, I had no idea what would happen to me. You get a picture in your head that's usually far worse than the real thing. In the last year I came to one of the pre-dialysis meetings and that was great. It was such a relief to see the treatments and talk to people who were dialysing.

George

Most kidney units now run pre-dialysis information groups, or 'seminars'. These can be very valuable for a variety of reasons. Firstly, they enable you to meet others who are in the same position as you. It is very easy to feel isolated by chronic illness and to believe that nobody else could possibly understand, or know what you are going through. It is also a chance for your spouse, partner or family to hear more about kidney failure and treatment. Partners often feel rather lost and excluded, because illness occupies so much of the patient's thoughts and energies. Those with kidney failure often fail to communicate their worries, and withdraw into themselves, which causes partners to feel anxious, useless and shut-out. Patients can also be irritable with other family members when they are feeling tired and generally low.

Another benefit of the information group is that you meet other members of the kidney unit team. This team does not consist just of doctors and nurses, but should include dietitians, counsellors or social workers, although this does vary throughout the UK. There may also be representatives of the local patients' association, who will give you the chance to find out what support and advice may be available for future use.

There may be a demonstration of peritoneal dialysis, and a chance to visit the haemodialysis unit. This enables you to talk to patients who are already coping well with the treatment, and to ask the sort of questions that you might not think of asking medical staff.

During the meeting, you will begin to see how the established patients, such as those who demonstrate the treatments, interact with their doctors and nurses. Some new patients are surprised to find that it is a very active and equal relationship, with the patient as a valued member of the team. In a lifelong condition such as kidney failure, hospital staff rely on people to take a lot of responsibility for their own health. The word 'patient' suggests somebody passive, but you need to be actively engaged in treatment. People often become real experts in managing their condition, and may know more about the treatment of kidney failure than their own GP.

Finally, there should be plenty of information about all aspects of the treatment.

Basic information about kidney failure

It is far easier to manage your condition if you understand what kidneys do, what happens when they stop performing as they should, and how treatments can replace the functions of normal kidneys. You may not want to take in all the information at once, but it can be useful to refer back to this section over the next few months.

Most of us are born with two kidneys, each about the size of our own clenched fist. The kidneys are found towards the back of your body, one on each side of the spine, tucked under the lower ribs, which protect them from injury.

Healthy kidneys are very efficient organs with a lot of reserve capacity. They do not have to work at full strength to do their job properly – in fact, one kidney is quite capable of doing all the work. This is why a healthy donor can give one of their kidneys to another person.

In most people with kidney problems, both the kidneys are more or less equally affected. You still may not notice that anything is wrong, because many people feel perfectly well until they have lost three quarters (75 per cent) of their function. At this stage, you are described as having 'kidney failure', although dialysis is not yet necessary. This explains why kidney failure is often diagnosed very late, as was the case for several of our contributors.

You may feel no symptoms, but a blood test would show that something is wrong. Even with advanced kidney failure, the urine you pass may look normal. But your doctor can tell from blood tests that there is a build-up of chemicals in the blood, which should have been passed out of the body by the kidneys. A blood test would show that you had raised levels of waste products (called creatinine and urea) in your bloodstream. If the level of creatinine in your blood is over 120 μmol/l (micromoles per litre of blood), then your kidneys are not working properly.

When 90 per cent of kidney function is lost, you are likely to feel ill — tired, breathless, itchy, sick and out of sorts. At this stage you will shortly need dialysis treatment to replace the work of the kidneys.

The table below gives a very rough guide to the progress of kidney failure, and suggests what you may expect. It must be stressed that people are all different and may not conform to 'standard' patterns. In addition, the cause of the kidney failure may affect how quickly it develops, and whether the progress of deterioration is 'in a straight line' or more 'stepwise' with little deterioration for a period, followed by another period of quite steep decline. It should also be remembered that not everyone with a creatinine level of, say, 500 μmol/l will feel the same. Treatment should be started when you feel begin to feel unwell, rather than when the creatinine reaches a particular level in your blood. Some people feel ill when their creatinine is 300–400 μmols/l. Others may still feel well with a creatinine of over 600, though they usually notice the improvement when dialysis is started!

A guide to diagnosis of kidney failure

Kidney function	Average time to dialysis	Symptoms	What will the doctor do now?
100%	very variable	No symptoms	Nothing
75%			Nothing
50%			Give you information
30%	Often within 1 year	Some (maybe)	Organise fistula (haemodialysis)
20%	3–9 months	Mild	Put in PD catheter (peritoneal dialysis)
10%	Any time from now, depending on symptoms	Moderate	Put on transplant waiting list and prepare for dialysis
5%	NOW!	Severe	Give dialysis (using fistula or PD catheter)

If kidney failure is diagnosed at an early stage, you may be able to carry on with damaged kidneys for months or even years before needing dialysis treatment, but it is unlikely the damage can be reversed.

What do normal kidneys do?

The most obvious function of the kidneys is to make urine. Urine contains waste products and any excess of chemicals and substances from our food which the body does not need. The kidneys filter these waste products from the blood, along with any excess water, and deliver the urine to the bladder to be passed out of the body.

If the body contains too much water – for example, through drinking more fluids than we need – normal kidneys are quick to filter out the excess and prevent the body becoming 'waterlogged'. Urine will be passed in large, rather dilute quantities, until the correct fluid balance in the body is achieved. If, on the other hand, the body is short of water (for example when we fail to drink enough, or in hot weather) the kidneys will conserve water by passing very little, highly concentrated urine.

By maintaining this balance, the kidneys control not only our water level, but also our blood pressure. Too much water in the system will put the pressure up, and too little will cause the pressure to drop too low.

The functions of healthy kidneys therefore include:

- **Constantly balancing the body's fluid** – to maintain a stable and correct level, neither dehydrated nor waterlogged.

- **Balancing the chemicals in the blood** – such as salt, potassium and phosphate which we absorb from our food, to maintain the best possible level of these substances.

- **Getting rid of waste products** – such as urea and creatinine, which are unwanted by-products of the activity of our muscles and the food that we eat.

- **Controlling blood pressure.**

The kidneys have two more important tasks:

- **Keeping the bones strong** – the kidneys have an important part to play in keeping our bones strong. To make strong bones we need a balance between calcium, phosphate and vitamin D. Healthy kidneys balance the calcium and phosphate levels needed to build bone, and convert the vitamin D in our diet into a form the body can use.

- **Stimulating the production of red blood cells** – to prevent anaemia. Healthy kidneys produce a hormone called erythropoietin. This hormone tells your bone marrow to produce more red blood cells whenever they are needed. These are the cells that give the blood its colour. Their job is to carry oxygen round the body.

If the kidneys are not working as well as they should, all these functions become less efficient. As kidney failure progresses, some people begin to notice symptoms.

Disturbed fluid balance
In kidney failure, when fluid balance is disturbed, the body may contain too much or sometimes too little fluid. If the body contains too much fluid, you may get swollen ankles and legs, puffiness round the eyes and in the hands. You may also feel breathless due to excess fluid in the lungs. If this happens, you may find it hard to lie flat at night and prefer to sleep propped up on pillows. Your blood pressure may be high.

If you have too little fluid, you may feel faint and giddy, especially when you get up suddenly from sitting or lying down. This is often because your blood pressure is low.

Build-up of waste products
When waste products, such as urea, start to build up in the body, you feel tired and 'off-colour'. You may lose your appetite and feel sick. You may go off sex. Waste products can also cause irritability, or loss of concentration and mental alertness. You may not notice these symptoms, but relatives and friends may be aware that you are less 'bright' than you were. Indeed many patients only realise how poorly they were when they notice the improvement following the start of dialysis.

Build-up of chemicals
When the level of chemicals (such as phosphate) gets too high (because the kidneys are no longer getting rid of the excess from your food) you may suffer from dry, itchy skin. You are most likely to notice this at night, when you get warm in bed. Some people also get cramps, or twitchy, restless legs. All these problems can make it hard to sleep properly.

Anaemia

Most people with kidney failure become anaemic (i.e. their blood can no longer carry enough oxygen around the body) because they are not producing enough erythropoietin. Anaemia contributes to the feelings of tiredness and lethargy. If you are anaemic, you get breathless when you exert yourself, and your energy levels are low.

As kidney function gets worse, there will be other changes that you are not aware of because they cause no symptoms. The most important of these is raised blood pressure, which will need to be controlled to maintain long term health. You will also be unaware of early changes to the bones, due to the lack of usable vitamin D, and the absorption of too much phosphate from food.

A summary of frequently reported symptoms of kidney failure

Tiredness	Irritability
Poor appetite	Nausea and sickness
Headaches	Weight loss
Swollen ankles/legs	Breathlessness
Itching and dry skin	Restless legs and cramps
Poor concentration	Loss of sexual interest
Sensitivity to cold	Sleep problems

These are the sort of problems that may make you visit your doctor. You might have many of these symptoms or very few. High blood pressure often has no symptoms, but it would be quickly discovered by your doctor. It is also unlikely that you will have noticed a change in your urine, although tests would show that it was of 'poor quality' (i.e. lacking in concentration and waste products). They would also show the creatinine level in your blood to be high (see page 21).

Many of these symptoms, particularly tiredness and lethargy, were reported earlier by some of our contributors. Others said that they felt perfectly well, right up to the time when they needed dialysis. Indira, the patient who reported sickness and vomiting (usually a symptom suggesting that dialysis should start), was diagnosed very late indeed.

In the kidney unit, we try to start dialysis *before* a person feels really ill. Sometimes it is difficult to persuade people to do this, because they want to put off dialysis for as long as possible. This is obviously their choice – a patient cannot be forced to dialyse. However, while many people fear that dialysis will be a dreadful ordeal, to be postponed as long as possible, the reality is usually far better than they expected. The only real benefit of delaying until symptoms become unpleasant, is that the difference made by dialysis is then very obvious and dramatic. Those who start earlier, when they still feel pretty well, often say that they doubt whether they really needed to start at all. They may think the treatment makes little difference at first – though most agree that they are feeling much better once they have settled on dialysis.

Further information

Further information about what happens in kidney failure, and the treatments available, see *Kidney Failure Explained* by Andy Stein and Janet Wild, available from Class Publishing, London.

More detailed information can be found in *Kidney Failure: The facts*, by Stewart A Cameron, available from Oxford University Press, Oxford.

3
Treatment during the pre-dialysis period

Following diagnosis, the aim is to keep you as well and fit as possible, to make the most of your remaining kidney function, and to give you enough information to enable you to manage your condition with the help of the kidney unit staff. This means not only dealing with any immediate problems, such as fluid retention, itching and anaemia, but also preventing long-term complications of kidney failure. These include damage to the heart and blood vessels due to high blood pressure, and weakening of the bones. Long term problems may not seem important at the time, but it is the aim of your kidney unit to keep you in good health for the rest of your life. This means thinking ahead.

As the time for treatment gets closer, you will need to discuss which type of dialysis you would prefer, and make preparations for this by having 'dialysis access' created (see pages 33–7).

Medication

Once you have been diagnosed as having kidney failure, it is likely that the doctor will prescribe you several new drugs. Don't worry if these are different from the medicines or pills other people at your clinic are taking. Everyone is different. While most patients need to take some tablets, tests will show the doctors which ones in particular you need. Occasionally the blood results show that no tablets at all are needed, but this is fairly rare.

Common medications
The drugs most commonly prescribed are:

- **For the protection of the heart and circulation**
  - Blood pressure tablets (antihypertensives);
  - Water tablets (diuretics);
  - Cholesterol-lowering tablets (statins).

- **For the protection of the bones, and to reduce itching**
  - Active vitamin D (Alfacalcidol or Calcitriol);
  - Phosphate binders (Calcichew, Alucaps, Phosex, Renagel and many others).

- **For anaemia**
  - Erythropoietin (EPO – examples include Aranesp, NeoRecormon) to raise your haemoglobin level. This is given by injection.
  - Iron (ferrous sulphate).

Most people hate taking lots of pills, especially when they do not feel any immediate benefit. In fact, some tablets, especially blood pressure tablets, can have unwanted side effects. If this is the case, rather than just stopping the tablets, *tell your doctor*, who can change your medication.

There are a great number of different blood pressure tablets and it should be possible to find one that suits you. It is very important to prevent damage to the heart and circulation due to high blood pressure. Good blood pressure control may also slow down damage to your kidneys, and delay the need for dialysis.

Phosphate binders protect your bones by preventing excess phosphate from your food passing into your bloodstream. To do this, they have to be in the stomach when the food arrives, or very soon after you start eating. There is no point in taking them unless you eat something, and no point in taking them an hour after eating, when the food has left your stomach.

Attitudes to medication

Our contributors have differing attitudes to their drug regimes. Some are very careful to take everything correctly, with only an occasional slip-up, and will probably benefit in the long term. Others, like the following contributors, have a more relaxed attitude which they might regret later.

I hate taking drugs, but I do take them every day. Maybe not as strictly as I should – I sometimes forget my phosphate binders with food. I decided early on that I wasn't going to be a slave to my kidney failure. The doctor's job is to keep me as healthy as possible, and I decide how I'm going to live my life. I listen to them and take it all on board, but I do bend the rules a bit to what I want to do. That's what keeps me going.

Andrew

I am on three or four different tablets, but I'm afraid I quite often slip up and forget something. My husband is very good, and reminds me, especially about the phosphate binders with meals.

Indira

I am careful to take all my drugs. I wasn't right at the start. I was on so many phosphate binders that I hardly had room for my meals, so I didn't always take them all.

Jenny

I'm not on many drugs. Just a blood pressure tablet. Oh, and Aranesp once a week to keep my haemoglobin up. And iron. And something three times a week – what would that be? I'm not that good on the drugs! Actually I'm not sure I'm on the one you take with food. I take a calcium acetate in the morning – perhaps I should be taking it three times a day with meals. I don't know. My levels are all right, because I looked at them.

Robert

The last quote reflects a common response to tablet taking, especially early on. It really is important for your long term health to take the tablets prescribed. So do ask, ask and ask again if you are not sure what you should be taking when, or if you cannot see why they might be relevant.

It's far easier to know *what* to take, and *when*, if you understand *why*. It may be sensible to ask for a list of what you are on, with an explanation of what each pill does, so that you can manage them better.

Diet

Some people do not need to follow a special diet before going on dialysis. Others do. Once you start dialysis, a diet may still be necessary, but it may change a little. You may also be asked to restrict your fluid intake. Most people need to cut down on salt in the diet, because salt encourages the retention of fluid and therefore raises blood pressure.

A blood test will show if any chemicals such as potassium or phosphate are building up. It will also show whether your cholesterol is too high, and you need to cut down on saturated fats. Potassium is, in fact, the most immediately dangerous substance for kidney patients. Unfortunately it occurs in many foods and is high in a lot of those that we particularly like, such as chips and crisps. Worse still, it is high in chocolate and coffee (especially instant coffee). If your potassium level becomes very high, it can interfere with the rhythm of your heart, so it is important to know whether you need to restrict it in your diet. Ask your consultant, and make an appointment to see your dietitian.

People who are approaching the need for dialysis often suffer from poor appetite, and can lose weight and become badly nourished. Your dietitian's aim, therefore, will be to see that you are eating enough food, of the right sort for you, to stay healthy.

I remember the dietitian came to see me when I was on the ward. I'd lost weight and had a very poor appetite so I said to her 'One thing I'm grateful for, is that you are not going to hit me with a diet, are you?' And she was so apologetic! I think she must have been sensitised by lots of bad reactions from people, because she apologised all the time. I must say that when she told me 'no chocolate or coffee . . .' that was hard to take! The diet was made easier at first by the fact that my urea was high, so I didn't feel hungry anyway.

Rhys

Very early on, I decided to swap potatoes for coffee. I didn't need to cut out all high potassium foods, so I chose just one as a luxury. You can't give up everything you like – not if you want to stick to the diet long term.

Jenny

In the past, dietitians were less flexible in their advice – which didn't always help patients to follow the guidelines, and certainly did little for their quality of life. Fortunately, the thinking on this important topic has changed, and dietitians will now try very hard to help you work out what is right for you as an individual. Just because you have kidney failure doesn't mean you shouldn't enjoy your food; indeed it is very important that you should be encouraged to eat well and maintain good nutrition.

What annoyed me about the diet is that I was given a long list of things I shouldn't eat. What I wanted to know was what I could eat. That was at the other hospital, where I first started dialysis. I'm much happier now, because my new dietitian is very positive, and shows me how to eat safely, without giving up all the things I like.

Chris

In the 1980s dietitians were not at all supportive, they were like the 'food police'. It was all what you couldn't do. I was so hungry! All the TV ads were for things I couldn't have. I recently asked to see the dietitian, and it was so different. They came with a list of 'negotiated foods', things you could have occasionally or swap for other things. I found I could have been having all the things I would have liked all those years, provided I was careful!

Jenny

The way in which your dietitian approaches the whole topic of food is very important. Nobody likes to be told that they can't have the things they enjoy eating, so a positive and flexible attitude is a real incentive to help you eat well and safely.

The diet has not really been a problem. Initially I followed all the instructions to the letter. But now, after six months on treatment, I know how to adapt it. I had to cut out milk products at first, but now it is everything in moderation. I have Indian food – curries, with lots of vegetables, balanced with some meat. My potassium is quite low, so I have been told I can be a bit less strict.

Indira

I like my food. I try not to eat the things I shouldn't, but I tend to eat a little of what I fancy and hope for the best.

Reg

I'm not cavalier about the diet. I find it's a matter of mental discipline. I say to myself, I don't need those things, and therefore I won't have them.

Rhys

Not everyone has this much self discipline. Frances sums up the way in which an experienced patient learns to manage the renal diet.

It's all a question of balancing it up. When you know what you're doing, you can allow yourself little treats and make up for them elsewhere. At Christmas they give you a recipe for a low potassium Christmas pudding, but I preferred to have a very small helping of the real thing. I have the occasional packet of crisps but I've given up peanuts, and I avoid very spicy foods because they make me thirsty. If I'm really craving chocolate, I have a chocolate covered wafer finger.

Frances

The more experience you gain, the better you will be able to manage this 'balancing-up'. It becomes second nature in the end. Jenny, who has had two decades of experience on dialysis, admits to being a 'real foodie', but says that when she first picks up a menu in a restaurant, she sees a 'list of chemicals'. She quickly eliminates the worst choices, then 'negotiates' the rest of the menu. If the main course is high in potassium, she chooses a low potassium second course, and vice versa. It is all a matter of practice.

• See your dietitian, and work out what you *can* eat.

Assessment for transplantation

If you are reasonably fit, and want to have a kidney transplant, you will be considered for the operation, even if you are over 70 years of age. Younger patients may be encouraged to go on the transplant waiting list before they need dialysis.

Once you have been accepted as a candidate by the transplant surgeon, certain details will be entered on a computer. These include information about your blood group and tissue type (which reveals your genetic make-up and so will help find the best possible 'match' for you). Whenever a donor kidney becomes available, your details will be compared with those of the donated kidney. The patient whose blood group is compatible with that of the donor, and whose tissue type is the closest match will be called in for final tests before receiving the transplant.

It is, therefore, not a queue that you are joining, but a sort of lottery. You might have to wait for several years before you get a good match, or you could be lucky the day after going on the list. Kidney transplants now have a high rate of success, but even well-matched kidneys last, on average, for only eight to ten years. This is an average. Some transplants fail in the early days, usually due to acute rejection by the body; others last for 20 years or more. Following the failure of a transplant, you can return to dialysis treatment. Provided you are fit enough for the surgery, you can receive a second, or even a third transplant.

If you have a well-matched living donor who is a blood relation, or even one (such as a husband or wife) who is not, the transplant can be planned in advance. Kidneys from living donors have the best success rate, because they do not have the trauma of being kept cold for several hours after removal, or transported long distances before being reconnected to the blood supply of their new host. The two operations, removal from the donor and transplantation into the recipient, take place at the same time, in adjoining operating theatres.

A common reason for a transplant to fail, is 'rejection'. This means that your body's immune system (which normally protects you by attacking invading bacteria), identifies the kidney as something that does not belong there naturally, and attacks it. To prevent this response, you have to take powerful medication to suppress your immune system. The drawback of this medication is that you are then less well protected against other 'foreign bodies' including bacteria and viruses, and are therefore at greater risk from infection.

The drugs to prevent rejection (called immunosuppressants) have to be taken for as long as you have the transplanted kidney. You will be on high doses at first, but these can be gradually reduced as the new kidney gets established, which should mean any drug side effects are also reduced.

Transplantation is an excellent treatment for many kidney patients, but long-term dialysis can provide a good alternative for those who are not suitable, or who simply do not wish to receive a transplant. It should be noted that life expectancy is approximately the same, whether you are on dialysis or have a transplant.

Further information
For more information about healthy eating if you have kidney failure, see *Food With Thought*, produced by the National Kidney Federation in conjunction with Amgen. Available from the NKF.

4
Types of dialysis treatment

Haemodialysis

Most people know about the haemodialysis machine, since publicity about kidney failure usually shows pictures of this sort of dialysis. The machine is quite large, and looks very complicated. Its job is to pump your blood through the system, ensuring that the temperature is maintained, the pressures are correct, that there are no leaks, or air in the system: in short, that all is safe. If this machine detects any problem, it stops – so it is failsafe. The actual 'artificial kidney', which cleans the blood as a healthy kidney would do, is called a 'dialyser'. It is attached to the side of the machine. A dialyser is a cylinder about a foot long and two inches across. It contains hundreds of tiny, threadlike tubes, through which your blood is passed. Meanwhile, dialysis fluid is pumped through the dialyser, washing the outsides of these tiny tubes. Tiny though they are, the tubes have microscopic holes in them – too small to let a blood cell escape, but large enough for the chemicals, waste products and excess water to be drawn out and washed away.

After three or four hours on the machine, all your blood will have passed through the dialyser several times, and will have been well cleaned. Dialysis usually takes place in hospital, either in the morning, afternoon or evening, on a regular rota, two or three times a week. Some people choose to perform their haemodialysis at home, which gives them far greater flexibility and cuts out a lot of travelling and waiting time. However, you do need a spouse, partner or other helper to be with you, or at least within earshot, while you are on the machine in case you need any help. People who want to work full time find it easiest to dialyse in the evening, either in hospital or at home.

Access for haemodialysis
In order to get your blood to the dialyser you need a fistula made at your wrist or elbow, or a soft plastic catheter inserted in your chest, just below your collar bone. These procedures are usually done under local anaesthetic, and are referred to as 'dialysis access'.

Fistulas

A fistula needs to be made several weeks in advance of dialysis, to allow time for it to heal and develop.

Creating a fistula involves making a join between an artery and a vein above your wrist. The blood in the artery, which lies *deep* in the wrist, is *fast-flowing*, because it is being pumped at high pressure by the heart. The blood in the vein, which lies *near the surface* of the skin, flows *slowly*, on its way back to the heart. The aim of the operation is to divert some of the fast-flowing arterial blood into the vein, to make it stand up on the surface of the skin. This makes it possible to insert two hollow needles into the vein, one to take blood to the machine, and one to return it to the body.

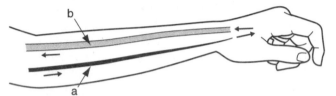

1. Blood is fast flowing in the artery (a), and slow moving in the vein (b)

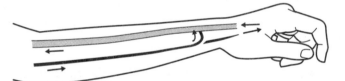

2. Some of the fast flowing blood from the artery is diverted into the vein to make it stand up on the surface of the skin

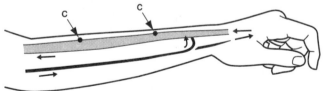

3. Two hollow needles can now be inserted into the raised vein at point 'c', one to take blood to the dialysis machine, one to return it

How a fistula works

A fistula is the best long-term access for dialysis, because it does not involve putting any plastic tubing into the body. Substances such as plastic can cause infection if left in the body. Once the operation site is healed, a fistula does not need a permanent dressing. After each dialysis, patients may have a pressure dressing put on until any bleeding stops, but the fistula is left uncovered for the majority of the time.

A local anaesthetic cream can be applied to the arm shortly before dialysis, before inserting the needles. After a few weeks, you may stop needing the cream, because the skin of the arm over the fistula begins to lose sensation.

Haemodialysis line

If your veins are not suitable for a fistula, you may be given a semi-permanent dialysis catheter (sometimes referred to as a Tesio catheter). This involves inserting a double-ended plastic catheter into an artery in the chest. The catheter emerges below the collar bone and remains in place between treatments, so it needs a dressing. There is no need for needles, because the dialysis lines are connected to the ends of the catheter as shown in the illustration. You might feel that this is a far better option than having a fistula, but this type of access has some disadvantages. Infections of the access site, (the place where the plastic lines enter the body), are fairly common. There is a risk of infection passing into the bloodstream along the plastic line, which can cause more serious illness. A dialysis line is not so reliable as a fistula in the long term, and is usually used for a limited time.

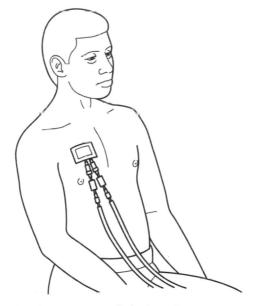

Semi-permanent dialysis catheter in situ

Peritoneal dialysis

Fewer people are aware of peritoneal dialysis, a treatment that is based at home. It involves draining dialysis fluid into your abdomen to absorb waste products, which can then be drained out again. You may often hear peritoneal dialysis referred to as 'PD'.

Access for peritoneal dialysis

Access for this type of dialysis involves placing a soft plastic tube, sometimes called a 'Tenckhoff catheter', into the abdomen. This tube will be about 30 cm (12 inches) long and about half of it will be positioned inside your abdomen, while the other half will be outside. Putting the tube into position can be done during a quick and simple operation, for which you are usually admitted to hospital overnight. It is usually done under a general anaesthetic, although it is possible to do it under a local anaesthetic. Techniques vary from unit to unit, but the tube is likely to come out below the navel and a few inches to one side or the other. Remember to let your doctor know which side will be most convenient for you. If you tend to

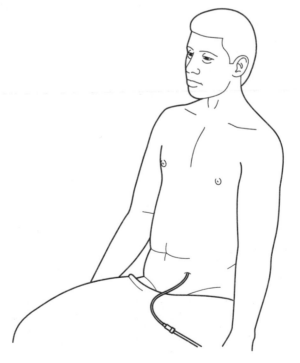

PD catheter in situ

sleep on your right side the catheter is more suitable on the left and vice versa. The soft plastic tube that comes from the abdomen ends in a sealed connector. The part that is inside your body lies in the peritoneal cavity, a space that contains your abdominal organs. This space is lined with a delicate membrane known as the peritoneum, a thin tissue with a rich blood supply.

Once the catheter has healed into place, dialysis fluid can be passed through the tube into the peritoneal cavity, where it lies in contact with the lining membrane. The fluid does not go into the stomach or bladder, or any of the organs inside you, but surrounds them, and fills up the gaps between them. Dialysis fluid generally comes in 2-litre plastic bags. It is composed of a sugar solution and additional chemicals, which draw waste products and excess water out of the bloodstream through microscopic holes in the membrane. Some of the chemicals enter the body as well (this is meant to happen). The fluid never comes into contact with your blood.

After bathing the membrane for several hours, the fluid containing the waste products and excess water can be drained out through the catheter, and fresh fluid is then passed in to continue the process. This is known as an 'exchange', since the used fluid is 'exchanged' for fresh fluid on each occasion. It takes 20–40 minutes and is a very gentle and continuous form of dialysis. Exchanges should be done four times a day, at reasonable intervals (so that each bag of fluid has several hours to bathe the peritoneal cavity and absorb waste products). This type of dialysis is known as 'CAPD', which stands for 'Continuous Ambulatory Peritoneal Dialysis'. 'Ambulatory' simply means that the process goes on while you walk around, carrying on your usual activities.

Automated peritoneal dialysis (APD)

When you have mastered the exchanges, you may be offered the automated peritoneal dialysis (APD) machine. Indeed, some areas have the appropriate resources to offer APD as an option straight away, however this is not the case in all parts of the UK.

The APD machine is set up beside your bed, and performs a number of exchanges, during 8–10 hours overnight, while you sleep. It is usually necessary to do one additional exchange using the manual technique already described for CAPD, during the day (at around teatime), but the rest of the day is free. This can be a very suitable treatment for someone who is at work, since it is sometimes difficult to take time off to do a CAPD exchange in the middle of the day.

Choice

Ideally, every person should be able to choose which type of dialysis they would like, having considered how it would suit their personal feelings, home and work commitments and preferred leisure activities. This does not always happen, for a number of reasons:

- Very late referral, when there is no time to plan which type of treatment will best suit the patient's lifestyle. (However, once established on dialysis, patients should have an opportunity to change therapy.)

- In some areas, hospital haemodialysis programmes may be full – making PD (which is performed at home) the only option. This may be used as a temporary solution if the patient would really prefer haemodialysis, which is offered when a place becomes available.

- There may be medical reasons which make one or other treatment more suitable.

Reasons why peritoneal dialysis may be unsuitable

If you are tall and muscular or overweight, it may be difficult to obtain adequate dialysis from PD. This form of dialysis tends to suit smaller men and women, though newer techniques mean this problem is reducing. It can also be difficult or impossible to establish PD if you have had several previous operations to the abdomen. These may have damaged and scarred the delicate peritoneal membrane, sticking it together in places. A damaged peritoneal membrane cannot filter the waste products efficiently.

PD may be hard to manage if you have severe arthritis or weakness in the hands. Very poor eyesight can also make it hard to do the exchanges neatly, without contaminating the connector. There are, however, special gadgets available to help partially sighted or blind people. Many blind people do PD very well, especially if they have a sighted partner who is willing to help them. If you have a hernia, you may need to have it repaired before attempting PD. If it cannot be repaired, then PD is not advised.

Reasons why haemodialysis may be unsuitable

If your blood vessels are very small, it may be hard to create a good fistula in the arm to take blood to the machine.

Haemodialysis removes excess water and waste products quickly over a short time. This can cause strain on the heart, so will not be advisable if you have a weak heart or have suffered from heart failure.

Freedom to choose

Our contributors had a variety of experiences with regard to choice. Some were involved in the decision making. Others, like Indira, were not.

> *I would have liked to have been given a choice, or to have been able to talk to somebody on treatment, but I was diagnosed so late. There was no time for planning. I was simply told that I would be having CAPD. I had no idea what was involved. When I found out, I was amazed that it was so simple.*
>
> **Indira**

It is often difficult for a patient to make a choice about treatment if they do not have enough information to enable them to plan what is best for them. The National Kidney Foundation's website features (among other useful items) a list of questions a patient should ask their doctor. This and other pages on this site will help you to explore which type of dialysis might be best for your particular circumstances.

> *I was given a choice. One of the things I had been dreading, when I knew that I needed dialysis, was the needles. The machine is the only thing you think of. I'd seen it on telly. I told the doctor I would almost prefer to die than to go through that process with needles on haemodialysis. Then I found out about the peritoneal dialysis, and I thought – 'Yes, I can handle that'.*
>
> **Rhys**

> *I was just told that I was too big to do well on PD, so I accepted that it would have to be haemodialysis.*
>
> **Robert**

> *I was given the choice, but I really couldn't be doing with PD exchanges four times a day. I didn't fancy that at all, so I opted for the haemodialysis machine.*
>
> **Mary**

Unfortunately, the 'choice' is sometimes one that is resource driven, and not what the patient might prefer at all.

> *I wasn't given a choice, because there was no room on the haemodialysis programme at my hospital at first. It was PD or nothing. It didn't really*

*suit my job, which is gardening, lots of heavy lifting and working with soil.
Later I changed to haemodialysis.*

Chris

Jenny, who has been on dialysis longer than any of our contributors
(24 years), tells us what the situation was like in 1980. She had a traumatic start to treatment. After only two sessions of haemodialysis, she was
given a transplant, but unfortunately the new kidney never worked properly. When the transplant failed three months later, she returned to the
hospital expecting to go back on haemodialysis. What followed shows how
much 'fight' and determination she has.

*They said, 'You're not having haemodialysis, you are having peritoneal
dialysis'. I said 'I'm not, I was on haemo before my transplant'. The doctor
said, 'What makes you think you have an automatic right to go on haemo?'
I said, 'But nobody has ever even mentioned peritoneal dialysis to me'.*

*He had his feet on the desk. I said, 'Get your feet off your desk when you
are talking to me!' Then he said, 'If you don't accept what we are offering,
you will die'. And I said, 'Alright, I'll die, but I'll make a lot of noise about
it!' I got my MP on to it. And, lo and behold, the next day I got my haemo
machine!*

Jenny

Happily, this sort of confrontation is seldom, if ever, necessary nowadays.

Pros and cons of the two treatments

It may be useful to look at the differences between the two treatments, to
work out which will fit better into your life, causing least disruption.

Time

The most tiresome thing about any dialysis treatment is the time involved.
There is not a lot to choose between *actual treatment time* for peritoneal
and haemodialysis, whether at home or in hospital. The chief difference
lies in the time travelling and waiting when you come in for hospital
haemodialysis. On PD, you will not need to visit the hospital often, perhaps
once every two months.

- CAPD – involves four exchanges, each taking around 20–40
  minutes depending on how experienced the person doing the

exchange is, and how quickly fluid drains in and out of their tummy. The exchanges should be spread through the day, and they have to be done every day. So (with preparation time) the exchanges take up 14–16 hours a week.

- **The overnight APD machine** – involves 8–10 hours per night, every night, but since you would have been asleep for most of this time in any case, it it hard to count it as time lost. Setting up the APD machine and disposing of the used fluid in the morning, accounts for about an hour per day, and you will probably need to do one manual exchange at teatime. If you discount the time you are asleep, the total is similar to CAPD.

- **Haemodialysis in hospital** – allows you four (sometimes five) dialysis-free days a week, which is obviously a major benefit. On dialysis days, you need to allow travelling and waiting time, which should be added to the 3–4 hour dialysis sessions. Travelling time may be very short, depending on distance, especially if you are able to drive yourself to and from treatment. If you depend on ambulance transport, the time increases considerably. Some patients complain that dialysis has taken up most of the day, due to transport delays, and the need to be ready and waiting for the ambulance well in advance. In addition, preparation for haemodialysis (including blood pressure and weight monitoring) takes about 20 minutes, and a similar length of time is needed to come off the machine and wait for bleeding to stop. Those who drive themselves may only devote 12–15 hours per week to treatment. Those on ambulance transport can spend 20 hours or more.

Freedom to travel

CAPD is a very portable system. If you want to go out for most of the day, the equipment for one exchange will fit into in a small sports bag. For a long weekend away, everything can be taken in the boot of a car. If you want to spend more time away, on holiday or business trips, you can have the dialysis fluid delivered to your destination, both in the UK and abroad. But you will need to ask the supplier at least four weeks in advance. The APD machine comes in a case the size of a weekend suitcase, which has wheels for easy transportation.

Haemodialysis is not quite so easy to arrange. Obviously you can go away for one or two days, since your dialysis schedule contains a 2–3-day break. To go away for longer, it is necessary to book into a hospital or dialysis facility near your destination. In the UK, most hospital programmes are very crowded, but there are a number of holiday dialysis centres, some on the sites of holiday camps, others near tourist centres on the coast. You should not need to pay for holiday dialysis in the UK.

If you want to travel abroad, there may be greater choice of dialysis centres and less pressure on dialysis spaces than in the UK. Within the European Community, you can dialyse using the E111 holiday medical insurance form and will not be charged for dialysis treatment. In the United States, it is still necessary to pay, and you may be charged £150 or more for a dialysis session. To find out details of dialysis centres in any part of the world, you can use the Globaldialysis website (see details on page 140).

Diet and fluid restriction

A large build-up of fluid puts a strain on the heart and circulation and raises blood pressure, so you will be asked to restrict the amount you drink.

When you start dialysis, you are likely still to be passing some urine. This helps to remove some of the excess water, even if the urine is of 'poor quality' (i.e. does not contain the waste products that it should.). At this stage, your kidneys are probably down to between 10 and 5 per cent of their normal function. The kidneys continue to decline over time. By 18 months or two years after starting dialysis, they are likely to be producing no urine at all. This means that *all* of your excess fluid has to be removed by dialysis.

On haemodialysis, excess fluid and waste products are only removed 2–3 times a week so, in between treatments, they can build up to high levels. To prevent this, you will be asked to restrict fluid intake, and follow a diet to maintain safe levels of potassium and phosphate.

On CAPD, fluid and waste products are being removed continuously, and never allowed to build up excessively. The fluid and dietary restrictions are therefore slightly less strict than for haemodialysis.

What can go wrong?

With CAPD and the APD machine, the most common problem is an infection of the lining of the abdomen (the peritoneum). This is called 'peritonitis'. On average, a patient will get an infection once every 18 months or two years. Since this is an *average*, some will get far fewer infections and others will get more. Most infections are mild, quickly diagnosed and treated, and cause little discomfort. If the infection is neglected, however, it can cause a painful illness, and damage the peritoneal membrane.

Peritonitis can be caused if you are careless while performing the exchange. For example, you may accidentally touch the end of the connector while it is open, allowing bacteria from your skin, or something you have touched, to travel down the catheter and cause infection.

Avoiding infections is a matter of careful and clean technique – and a bit of luck. If you suspect that you have contaminated the connector, you should ring and talk to your PD nurse immediately rather than wait to see what happens. You will probably be prescribed an antibiotic to prevent the problem before it can start.

Complications for haemodialysis patients are usually due to the dialysis access (see pages 33–5). Sometimes the flow becomes restricted, and not enough blood can be taken from your veins to the machine. You may need to have your access 'revised' – moved to a different place on your arm, or to the other arm, involving another operation.

Patients having haemodialysis can also contract infections. Those with a fistula are unlikely to have many such problems, but those with a dialysis catheter may get bacteria travelling down the line into the bloodstream. Treatment is with antibiotics. If the infection is bad, you may need to have the catheter replaced or moved.

Two types of dialysis: a summary of pros and cons

	Haemodialysis	PD
Effectiveness	Virtually always adequate	May not be adequate
Time	15–20+ hours per week	14–16 hours per week
Travel	Possible but needs planning	Comparatively easy
Work	Possible. Evening dialysis if full time	Comparatively easy
Fluid	Pretty strict	Less strict
Diet	Pretty strict	Less strict
Complications	Mostly access modifications; infections	Peritonitis infections
Daily life	Can be 'left behind' at hospital	You are in control

Home haemodialysis

Some patients may wish to consider having haemodialysis at home, allowing them to schedule their treatment when it is most convenient. If this is an option, the hospital will pay for the machine and installation at home. Patients likely to receive a transplant within a short period of time would not be considered for home training. However, if a transplant is unlikely, and the patient is well established and stable on dialysis, it may be a good option.

If you want to do haemodialysis at home, you need to have a partner, friend or family member willing to be with you during treatment, to ensure that all is well, and to contact the hospital if help is needed.

You and your helper will be trained at the hospital in the use of the machine. This will take a number of weeks before you are ready to start home treatment. Once you are both confident, you will start dialysing at home. One of the unit nurses will attend the first home treatment to ensure all is going well. The hospital will install a telephone beside the machine, so that you can ring the unit if you have any difficulties.

There are obvious advantages in having your dialysis at home. You do not have to travel to hospital. You can dialyse when it is most convenient for you, and there is no waiting around.

Home haemodialysis won't suit everybody, however. Some people prefer to keep all evidence of their kidney failure out of the home and only be reminded of it when attending hospital. Others find it a strain on their relationship to involve their partner in the treatment, and the partner has to make a considerable commitment of time. It is sometimes better if two family members or friends are able to learn to help the dialysis patient, because each can give the other a break from time to time.

Jenny dialyses at home, and describes her treatment:

I think the pros outweigh the cons. Because I dialyse at home, I am my own boss. There's nobody to nag me about what I should and shouldn't do. I always meditate for a while before going on, to relax me, which I couldn't do in hospital. Then I can ring my friends and watch videos during dialysis. I always give myself a treat of toast and peanut butter during the early part of treatment, because I love it, but it's high in potassium. That means it gets 'dialysed out' later in the treatment. I also think it's good not to have to 'put on a face' for the staff and other patients. If I'm down, or in a bad mood, I can show it.

The biggest thing against it is the strain it puts on my husband. He gets upset having to see me on the machine. Another thing is that you forget that there are lots of others in the same situation. I hardly ever meet a dialysis patient – all my friends are fit and well. It makes me feel a bit different, isolated, and I sometimes think 'nobody really understands'. I can get like a spoilt brat. When I do visit the unit, I see people far worse off than me and feel ashamed.

Jenny

If home haemodialysis suits you and goes well, it is probably the best long-term dialysis treatment, providing a good quality of life and flexibility to do the things you want to do.

These, then, are the options. Some people swear by peritoneal dialysis, others by haemodialysis. There are many people who try both types of treatment at different times during their lives.

Further information

The National Kidney Federation's website www.kidney.org.uk contains a medical information zone including information and slideshows about haemodialysis and peritoneal dialysis.

The leaflets *Introduction to Haemodialysis* and *Introduction to Peritoneal Dialysis*, published by the National Kidney Federation, are available from the NKF, full details on page 141.

5
Starting dialysis

Putting it off

It is very common for people to try to put off starting dialysis. There is never a good time, it seems. Certainly not for Rhys or Indira.

I strongly suspect that they wanted me to start straight away when I was diagnosed in September, and in hindsight that might have been a better thing. But at the time I wanted to avoid dialysis. I had also booked a dream holiday in America, with my son, in October. And I wasn't going to let anything interfere with that. So we went on holiday; and then there was too much going on in my work at the school, so I waited till the end of term. I decided to use the Christmas holidays to get myself sorted out.

Rhys

When they told me my kidneys had failed, they wanted me to start dialysis then and there. I suppose I should have started immediately. But I felt so much better after starting water tablets to get rid of all the fluid which was making me breathless, that I thought I could carry on. Besides, I was in the middle of changing my job, so it was a bad moment, so I put it off for a few weeks.

Indira

Some patients, like George and Robert however, find it easier to start dialysis as soon as they can, so that they can feel more in control of what is going on.

I didn't try to put it off. I said to the consultant, whatever you'd do for yourself, that's what I want for me. I started when he decided it was the right time.

George

I didn't want to start as an emergency. If you start in a controlled fashion you feel better. We talked to the staff and they talked to us and we worked our own game plan out.

Robert

Our contributors did not all have an easy start to treatment, and the benefits were not instant. Those who are determined sometimes expect too much of themselves too quickly when they start dialysis. You need to allow time to adjust, as starting dialysis is likely to be a milestone, in both physical and mental terms.

I spent a week in bed when I first came home after having the catheter in to start CAPD. My husband said to me, 'you can sit there for ever if you like, and become a vegetable, or you can get on with it.' He got me moving. It was a bit painful at first because the stitches were pulling, and everything was a bit foreign, what with the tube in my tummy. I was frightened to move. And when I got out of bed, he said 'straighten up!'. He bullied me, but it worked. I was out shopping the next week, and within a month I was back at work. I didn't notice much difference when I first started CAPD, except for my skin. That had been so dry and itchy I could hardly bear it, and that improved after a few days. I also had very swollen ankles, I could hardly get my shoes on, and they gradually went down.

Frances

I had a bad time to start with. There were problems for me with CAPD. I wasn't getting enough dialysis, and the four exchanges seemed to dominate my life. I kept looking at my watch, thinking how much time I had before the next exchange. I was back at work, trying to fit it round everything else. The whole thing was ruling my life. So I changed to the overnight treatment [APD]. I had been warned that it would take a while to feel the benefits of dialysis, which was good because I had thought I'd feel better instantly. After three months I felt a lot better.

Rhys

As these quotes show, you may need to be a bit patient with yourself when starting treatment. Like Frances, you may lack confidence at the start, and need encouragement to 'get you going'. Dialysis staff sometimes stress how much better you will feel when you dialyse – knowing that, before long, this will be true. It can however be a disappointment when you do not feel better immediately. This is especially true if you have started treatment in good time, before you feel really ill.

> *I felt well before starting dialysis, so didn't notice a lot of difference at first. I was still going to the gym and that sort of thing. I started because my potassium and phosphate levels were getting high. I have noticed that I have more energy now. If I go on a day trip with the kids, I don't get tired like I used to.*
>
> **George**

> *I didn't feel better immediately when I started haemodialysis, but I wasn't too bad beforehand in any case. It took about six weeks to notice that I really felt better. I wasn't getting so tired.*
>
> **Mary**

> *Patience is important. I wanted to overreach myself too early and pretend that everything was normal, but I was carrying on a façade of normality. I should have cooled off a bit and let myself recover.*
>
> **Rhys**

At first, the new regimes you have been taught may seem daunting. It's like learning any new skill – for example, driving a car. At first you have to think very hard about using the brake, clutch and accelerator in the right order, but later it becomes second nature. The same is true of dialysis.

> *When I started, I was on CAPD. I found I had so many words and instructions from the nurses running round in my head, it was like being re-programmed. I felt that the life I had before took second place and everything was diverted into dialysis. So I thought, I may be a renal patient but I need other things in life, chiefly my work. I will find ways to fit dialysis round my everyday life.*
>
> **Chris**

A summary of what to expect when starting dialysis

Haemodialysis

It takes a while for the body to adjust to haemodialysis treatment. For the first few sessions, you may feel a bit lightheaded or headachy at the end of treatment. For this reason, it is better to have somebody drive you in and out of hospital for the first couple of weeks. As you become accustomed to dialysis, you should be able to drive yourself, which can save a great deal of time.

Some people feel 'washed out' following treatment, due to the removal of fluid. This usually gets better after a few hours.

If you had symptoms, such as nausea, breathlessness or itching, before starting dialysis, these should resolve over the first few weeks. If you thought that you had no symptoms, you may be surprised to find that you are feeling better, more alert mentally, and less tired.

Peritoneal dialysis

Even if you plan to have automated peritoneal dialysis (APD) in the longer term, many people start by learning to do CAPD exchanges four times a day. At first, these may seem to rule your life. You find yourself clock-watching. You may feel unsafe doing an exchange away from home, and therefore unable to exploit the flexibility of CAPD. As you become more practised at doing the exchanges, however, they will become easier. In time, you will find you hardly have to think about what happens next. After a while, you may be able to do them in odd places. (We have known long distance lorry drivers who do them in the cab!)

Initially, you may experience a little discomfort towards the end of draining out the fluid. This usually disappears after a week or two. Some people on CAPD find that they suffer from constipation. If this is a problem for you, do make sure you discuss it with your PD nurse.

As with haemodialysis, it may be a few weeks before you are aware of the benefits of the treatment. With both types of dialysis, many people find that once they have settled on treatment, they feel so much better that they can't understand why they didn't ask to start months earlier.

It was such a relief to me and my wife when I started dialysis. The uncertainty beforehand had been terrible, not knowing what it would be like. When I started, we could see what the worst was going to be, and plan round it. And it wasn't that bad at all.

George

When they showed me what was involved with CAPD, I felt happier. I had been thinking of a huge dialysis machine. This was so simple. I felt very unwell before I started, and I felt better fairly quickly. I didn't feel nearly so sick, although I am still sometimes sick in the morning – it only lasts a few minutes, then I get ready for work. People tell me I look really well now.

My hair is shinier and my skin is much better. I did the CAPD treatment for two or three months, then I was given the APD machine.

Indira

Further information

For more information about starting dialysis, see Chapter 5 of *Kidney Dialysis and Transplants: the 'at your fingertips' guide* by Andy Stein and Janet Wild, available from Class Publishing, London.

6
Kidney transplants: the choices

I know it's different for some people, but in my experience you survive on dialysis but you live with a transplant.

Keith

There is no doubt that a good kidney transplant allows the best possibility of a near normal life for some people with kidney failure. Dialysis only provides about 5 per cent of normal kidney function, which is enough to keep you alive and reasonably well. A good transplant provides 50 per cent of normal kidney function, which is enough to return your blood chemistry to normal levels. Most people find that their energy and wellbeing, including their capacity for sex and parenthood, are restored by transplantation.

Will a transplant be suitable for you?

As indicated on page 31, some people are assessed for transplantation before starting dialysis, and may even receive a donor kidney before they need to start dialysis treatment. (This is especially likely if they are having a kidney donated by a close friend or relative.) It is however, more common to consider transplantation after being established on dialysis. This has some advantages, in that you will be cushioned against future problems. You will have learned how to manage the system that is your safety net. If your transplant does not function, which is an unusual but possible outcome following the surgery, or if it fails after a number of years, you will simply return to dialysis – a way of life that you have already mastered. That is what happened to Laura.

When I started dialysis, I was on CAPD. I had a catering business, then I changed to massage and aromatherapy after I had my transplant. I did all the qualifying courses. I had a really good business. Last year when my transplant failed, I couldn't work for three months and lost a lot of clients. Now I'm on APD I am getting back into the swing, and building things up again.

Laura

Reasons for wanting a transplant

There are a number of pros and cons to consider, which you will be able to discuss with the staff of your transplant unit. Briefly, the pros are as follows:

- Many people feel very much better than they ever did on dialysis.

- You are free of the need for dialysis, and the restrictions on diet and fluid that go with it.

- It is much easier to get around – you can travel the world if you want to.

- Complications of kidney failure, such as bone disease, are prevented and may be partially reversed by transplantation.

- Fertility and sexual function usually return to normal, allowing you to have children if you wish.

Reasons to be wary of having a transplant

The cons, however, are quite considerable:

- You will need to take two or more immunosuppressant drugs to prevent your body rejecting the new kidney, including a steroid and a drug to combat those cells which attack any 'foreign bodies' they find in your system. If you fail to take these drugs, even for a couple of days at any time, your immune system will recognise the kidney as a foreign body and attack it, causing the transplant to fail.

- Side effects of these drugs may be quite severe in the early stages, causing changes in your mood, (which may be very 'up and down') and in the way you look. You may develop facial hair, and a swollen face as the result of the steroids. Some people complain of shakiness and tremor. Most of these effects decrease after the first six months, when your drug regime is gradually reduced to a maintenance dose.

- On some drug regimes, around 15 per cent of patients develop diabetes. This may be temporary in some cases, but a proportion of individuals will require lifelong insulin treatment.

- More serious problems can be caused by suppressing your immune system. These can include infections by certain viruses, which are normally attacked and killed by the white blood cells in your blood.

- There is also an increase in the occurrence of certain cancers as a result of this immunosuppression. Some are easily treated, such as skin cancers, which seldom invade the rest of the body. Others, such as lymphomas, can be life-threatening. It should be stressed that 95 per cent of transplanted patients do *not* get serious cancers as a result of these drugs; but it would not be honest to pretend that there is no increased risk at all.

A transplant kidney does not last for ever. On average, a kidney will last for 8–10 years, though kidneys from living donors tend to last longer.

If, following discussion with your doctors and nurses, you are found to be fit for the surgery and are still keen to receive a transplanted kidney, you will be placed on the transplant waiting list.

Not everyone is suitable for transplantation. If you are already frail, due to age or other illnesses, it may be too much of a risk to undergo major surgery. Others, who have worked out a way of living on dialysis that gives them a good quality of life may choose to remain on this form of treatment – particularly if they have already had one transplant fail.

I like being in control of things, and I wouldn't feel I was in control with a transplant. Things are not perfect but they are going OK and I don't want to rock the boat.

Jenny

Having had a failed transplant does not put everyone off the idea though. Paul manages on dialysis, but he would be delighted to be offered the chance for another transplant:

Another thing that keeps me going is the thought of getting another kidney. When that happens, it's funny, but you forget all about the time on dialysis.

Paul

Keith, who had an unhappy time with an unsuccessful first transplant, was wary of a second transplant at first, but later decided to go back on the waiting list.

After the first transplant, I didn't go straight back on the waiting list. It did affect me, the fact that it had failed. At first I wasn't prepared to go through it again – but then I decided to try once more, and it went well right from the start. It was all much easier second time around!

Keith

Transplants from living donors

Since the supply of donor kidneys from people who have died is limited, it may be months or even years before a suitable, well-matched kidney becomes available. With this in mind, more and more people are receiving a kidney from a living donor, usually a close relation. A parent, brother or sister is likely to have a similar tissue type to yours, and will therefore be 'a good match'. The drugs to prevent rejection have improved over the last few years, making it possible to use a less well-matched kidney successfully. This has made transplants between partners and close friends possible, indeed in some centres, such living unrelated donors are in the majority.

Transplantation from a living donor needs very careful thought. There are psychological as well as physical considerations to be taken into account.

If a parent gives a kidney to a son or daughter, it creates a very real psychological bond between the two. If the relationship is already a good, relaxed and non-possessive one, this need not be a burden to the person receiving the kidney (the recipient). The same may also be true if one spouse or partner donates a kidney to another. If however there are mixed or troubled feelings in the relationship, these can become high-lighted and emphasised by the donation of the kidney. If, as rarely happens, the kidney fails to function, or is rejected, the donor can also feel that they and their 'gift' have been rejected.

The problem, for some donors, is to stop seeing the kidney as belonging to them following the transplant. The recipient may feel that they have let the donor down, if the transplant fails. The same applies to donations between brothers and sisters, though the psychological bond is less complicated by issues of dependence. If, however, the donor is married, it is important to ensure that the spouse and family of the donor are willing and happy for the transplant to go ahead. There can be tangled family resentments which are triggered and come to the surface at the time of a living donation.

The risks to the donor's life, if they are in good health, are very small, but the removal of a kidney is always a major operation. Recovery time is sometimes longer for the donor than for the recipient, and some donors complain of persisting discomfort from the operation. Both will take about three or four months to return to work, so there are also financial considerations.

Personal experiences of kidney transplants

Since they were first interviewed for this book, two of our contributors, Robert and Indira, have received transplant kidneys. Both had had their new kidneys for about four months when I spoke to them again. Neither has had a completely trouble-free time since the operation, but both are now getting back to normal life. First they explain how they were called in for the operation:

It was 4.00 am when the telephone went, so I immediately thought something was wrong with someone in the family. Then they said they had a kidney for me. We packed a bag and drove in. I'd only been on the waiting list for 89 days! My feelings were muddled – excitement, anxiety, it was all a bit of a blur. On the way to the hospital, I was thinking 'we had snow yesterday, I wonder if someone was killed in a road accident and I am getting their kidney'. When we arrived I asked where the kidney had come from, and they said Portsmouth. So I imagined it came from a sailor.

Robert

My telephone call came at 1.30 am. I reacted with disbelief at first, I thought it was a joke. I had been in London on a course and was very tired. I really wanted to sleep, but I knew I had to go in. I hadn't packed a bag so I did that and we set off. When we got there they did a few tests, then said that as I had a slight cold they would not be able to do the operation. So I started packing again. But the surgeon came in and said that as it was a good match, he advised giving me antibiotics, waiting 6 hours, and then going ahead.

Indira

Both Robert and Indira were called in the middle of the night, which is a common time for patients to be told there is a transplant available. Robert showed great interest in where his kidney had come from. People often want to give their new kidney a 'background' so that they can carry on its 'life story' from the moment they receive it.

There is usually a longish wait while final tests are done, and the patient is dialysed if they need it.

Indira waited for six hours to make sure the antibiotics had started working before she was prepared for the operation. Robert, too, recalls 'twiddling his thumbs for several hours'. Then a nurse came to ask if he would take part in a trial of a new drug after the transplant, which he agreed to do.

I made phone calls to various people to let them know where I was. All the tests were done by midday. I was told to change, then I was told to rest till 2 pm, when they took me down to theatre. I had my pre-med, and I could see the surgeon through the window. I asked the nurse to ask him if I could see the kidney. I'd have liked to see it, but the surgeon wasn't happy with the idea. Next thing I remember, I woke up saying, 'I need a wee, I need a wee' so it must have been working! It was 6 o'clock in the evening. It all went so well, I was out of hospital in eight days.

Robert

Indira had a different experience:

The operation went smoothly, no problem. But the kidney didn't produce urine, I'm not sure why. They said it was a 'sleeping kidney'. I had haemodialysis while I was in hospital, and I had strong anti-rejection therapy and high doses of steroids, which unfortunately made me hallucinate. So they kept giving me short breaks in between, because I felt quite wiped out. They bombarded me with everything for three and a half weeks. I was literally begging them to let me go home, and they would say, maybe in a few days, then it would be maybe a couple of days more . . . It was so depressing because I would see people come in for their transplants and go home again, and I was still there. It all became sort of dreamlike.

Indira

Transplanted kidneys sometimes take a long time, even several weeks, to recover from the 'trauma' of being removed, kept cool for a period, then moved into a new host. This problem is called 'acute tubular necrosis' or ATN. The kidney may shut down for a while, but is able to recover with time and function well.

Robert started well, but then began to get some problems. Instead of returning to near normal, his creatinine stayed a little high.

Over the first four or five weeks things got better and better. Then I came to a sort of plateau, and things didn't go on improving any more. My creatinine is around 190–200. I've still got high blood pressure, my pulse is really fast, and I have got the shakes. It's all from the cocktail of drugs I'm on, though I am starting to reduce them. I'm on . . . well, you know me! I could never remember drugs. I seemed to be taking handfuls of tablets. I'm taking 20 tablets a day now. It was 34 at first!

Robert

Indira's kidney 'woke up' after eight weeks, and is now working well. With her usual optimism she says:

I met one woman who said she still needed dialysis for six months before her kidney woke up. So perhaps I was lucky.

Indira

Robert too is hoping for the best, but admits:

I'm a bit disappointed. It all started so well, but I would like to feel better than I am. I actually felt fitter on dialysis. I'd like to feel at least as well as I did on dialysis. Every day is an improvement though. Maybe other people don't feel so bad on the drugs. It's probably just me. I have said I'll go back to work tomorrow, because I want to move on, I want to make progress and get back in the swing of things. Once the drugs are reduced, I hope I'll feel OK. They have told me that the kidney may not be getting enough blood, so they are planning to do an angiogram to look at its blood supply, because my creatinine is still a bit high.

Robert

Indira, too, is eager to get back to work, having hoped to return after three months. Now she is planning to go back at five months. She has been through a considerable upheaval in her life in a very short time, and is wise to be patient with herself:

Everything has really happened so quickly. Less than a year ago I was diagnosed, I started dialysis in August, learned CAPD and then APD, went on the transplant list in December and at the end of January I was transplanted. I was lucky of course, but I never had a chance to settle at any time. Things are not stable yet. I have had four months with the transplant. I planned to get back to work by now, but I have put it off for one more month.

Indira

She has kept in close touch with her employers, and they are being very sympathetic:

I went to talk to them and they have agreed I'm not quite ready . . . I need to get my confidence back. I feel that everybody can see how bad I am. I am shy of meeting the people at work because I had never told them I had a kidney problem. Body image is a big problem for me, because my face is quite swollen with the steroids, and I feel people will stare at me. My supervisor knows everything, and she has suggested I come in and have a

*coffee with the team one day to break the ice. She has said I could start by
doing one day a week. I just need to face it.*

Indira

Keith agrees that getting back to work is an important part of recovery,
not only from the physical point of view, but because of the psychological
benefits:

*I think that when you have had a major operation like a transplant and are
off work for a while, you become inward-looking. You sit at home asking
yourself how you are feeling from moment to moment and noticing every
detail. The key is to get back to what you were doing before. That changes
your focus and then you won't be so aware of any side effects.*

Keith

When asked what difference the transplant had made to their lives,
Robert and Indira both pointed out that their problems made it impossible
to judge as yet. Both expected, quite realistically, to feel considerably better
within a few months, when the immunosuppressant drugs had been further reduced.

*The difference it has made is that I don't have to go for dialysis three times
a week. That's a big plus. I have been going to transplant clinic once a week
so far. But that is going to be two weeks from now on. I've been off work for
four months now. Perhaps I'm just being impatient. It's definitely the
drugs that are having this bad effect. I wake up feeling fine, but then I have
to take the drugs and the shakes start. I feel so well before I take them that
I almost forget them. I've put on weight too, but I am trying not to eat too
much.*

Robert

*I have only just started to feel the difference, because at first I felt bad with
the medication. To be honest, up until now I have felt I would rather have a
clear head and do dialysis than have the transplant. I feel so out of control
at the moment. Within minutes of taking my medication, I start shaking.
With dialysis, I was in control. I would start treatment regularly at 10.00
in the evening. I knew where I was, it wasn't painful, I controlled it. Now
there is no going back. I have the transplant, so I have to take the
medication, and I can't control the side effects.*

Indira

Keith remembers the early side effects from his second transplant, 17 years ago:

> *The ciclosporin makes you feel shaky when you are on a high dose, but it gets better as it is reduced. Yes – there is a whole list of problems that you might get from the immunosuppressant drugs, and the unit has to tell you about all of them – but most people only get one or two of them, and – come on! A bit of shakiness? It's better than dialysis three times a week!*
>
> **Keith**

Indira sums up the problem as she sees it, in terms of a loss of self-confidence. Her reaction to this was not to retire into herself, but to prove to herself that she is still able to work:

> *I think one of my problems is confidence. My medication is still high, so I am still shaky and I don't want anyone to see me. I know I can manage the work, because I have been doing reports for work from home. I have been interviewing people for a care agency and doing the reports, so I have been keeping myself going. I needed to do something. You can't just sit and watch television, and my concentration for reading has not been very good. I just needed to prove to myself that I could still do things. I found I had to read and re-read what I had written to make sure it made sense. My mind feels a bit fogged, but that is an effect of the drugs and will get better when they are reduced.*
>
> **Indira**

What is evident from these quotes, is that the same positive and determined spirit that made Robert and Indira cope so well with life on dialysis is still helping them through a difficult start to transplantation.

Most patients who have a transplant have an easier time than either of our contributors, and can feel real benefits at an earlier stage. Indeed, there are some who feel it is literally life-transforming, as Keith explains:

> *Basically, a transplant gives you your life back. I can come home from work and think, 'Now, do I want to go to the pictures, or to a night club, or out for a drink, or do I want to watch football on the TV?' I used to have no choice: I had to dialyse.*
>
> *It also enabled me to think about my career and to change my job. I joined the fire service, and started by taking the 999 calls. In the end I was*

promoted to Team Leader. Now I work as a Community Education Officer – talking to schools about safety.

My energy levels are better and I can eat and drink what I like. I can drink beer again! The key thing is that I can make choices again.

           Keith

Helen's story involves more then one person and more than one transplant!

I was on haemodialysis in hospital, and then I met Nick, who had recently had a transplant. I have diabetes and my kidneys failed when I was 25. We became good friends and he supported me, because he had been on dialysis and knew what it was like. About a year later I was called in for a transplant.

It took about two weeks for me to begin to feel better. I wasn't tired or bloated anymore and I had a lot more energy. Later he moved in with me and we became partners. Then, after he had had it for five years, Nick's transplant failed. We decided to have his dialysis at home. I learned how to help him with the haemodialysis machine, and we did it together. We both carried on working, but we managed to fit everything in somehow!

We got married last September, in a really lovely ceremony. Our best wedding present came in February this year, when Nick had another transplant. It has gone really well.

It has made a great difference to our love life. Lovemaking never used to enter his head when he was on dialysis, but now it is really good. We want a baby now. With his transplant going well, perhaps our luck has changed!

           Helen

Transplantation can be a very positive step for those who want to have a child, and cannot do so while on dialysis. But some are unable to have a transplant, or – like Jenny – would rather base their lives on the framework of regular dialysis. So it is comforting to know that patients can live long, full and successful lives while relying on dialysis alone.

Further information

For more detail about what the transplant operation involves, the benefits and implications of going for a 'living transplant' and how your life will be affected after the operation, see Chapters 11, 12 and 13 of *Kidney Failure*

Explained by Andy Stein and Janet Wild, available from Class Publishing, London.

More information about transplants can be found on the website of the UK Transplant Support Service (see page 143).

7
Building a relationship with the kidney unit

Kidney unit staff have a difficult job. They have to do their best to concentrate your attention on your treatment, giving diet and fluid advice and prompting you to take the drugs. Yet they should also be helping you minimise the effects of treatment on daily living, devoting as little time as possible to dialysis and encouraging you to lead a normal life. This can result in you receiving mixed messages, due to conflict between the two aims.

It is important that the relationship does not become 'parental', with the patient acting as a rebellious teenager, trying to get away with things. It is also important to try to avoid being a passive, disinterested recipient of treatment. The relationship can only work well if it is an equal and adult partnership, with respect on both sides.

> *Use the staff to your advantage. They are there to help. New patients, in particular, need a staff member to talk to. You need consistency and continuity. This is where your 'named nurse' comes in. After a while, she or he will understand how you tick, and will be able to tell if and where you are going wrong, and give you advice in the right way for you.*
>
> *Chris*

In some units, the patient sees their consultant nephrologist on a regular basis, but it is more usual to see a more junior doctor for many appointments. Your consultant will still be in overall charge of your case, and any problems will be referred to him or her for advice.

The people you will meet in hospital

As well as your kidney doctors, you will meet a number of specialist nurses who make up the kidney unit team. It varies between units, but your first contact with one of these specialists may be with the pre-dialysis nurse.

Pre-dialysis nurse

A pre-dialysis nurse's task is to assess your case as you approach the need for treatment, taking into account your physical condition, family commitments, job, housing and preferences. The pre-dialysis nurse may liaise with a social worker or counsellor, as well as the medical team, to help get a full picture of your case. You should get plenty of information about different treatments, and will be able to ask questions. Your pre-dialysis nurse may also be a link with pre-dialysis education services if your unit runs them.

Access co-ordinator

Many units also have an access co-ordinator (often a nurse), whose job is to assess your need for dialysis access, in particular for the creation of a fistula. The nurse will co-ordinate the whole process of referral until the operation has been successfully performed. The nurse will liaise with the surgical team to arrange the operation you need to make dialysis possible, and will check whether the result is satisfactory. You may need to have a 'revision' (a further operation) of your access if the blood flow is not good enough to provide efficient dialysis. Your fistula will be monitored regularly – it is the access nurse's responsibility to keep an eye on it and make sure that any problems are dealt with as quickly as possible. If you are having a fistula made, the nurse needs to check the blood vessels in your arm to see where the best blood flow can be obtained. The flow can be measured from the outside (without using needles) with a machine called a Doppler. After the operation, you should be able to feel a slight 'buzz' if you put your finger over the fistula. If the buzz stops, it may mean that the fistula is blocked by a clot, which should be treated immediately. You should contact your access nurse straight away if this happens.

Anaemia co-ordinator

As mentioned on page 24, kidney patients often have too few red blood cells to deliver enough oxygen and nutrients around the body. This is called anaemia and leads to tiredness and breathlessness. A blood test called the haemoglobin test (Hb) is used to monitor anaemia. If the level is below 11.0 g/dl, then you are anaemic and may need treatment with erythropoietin (EPO). EPO is a hormone made by normal kidneys in order to stimulate the production of more red blood cells, but now available in replacement form which is given by injection once or twice a week.

The anaemia co-ordinator (again, usually a nurse) is part of the team in many renal units and helps to monitor your Hb. The anaemia co-ordinator will be involved with decisions about if and when you need to start EPO and what the correct dose should be for you (it is very variable). You will also need checks on your iron levels as iron is needed to make red blood cells. EPO cannot work if you do not have the right building materials for blood in your body.

Haemodialysis nurses

If you are on haemodialysis, your named haemodialysis nurse will be a very important person in your life. The task of the haemodialysis nurse is to attach you safely to the machine, monitor your dialysis, and ensure that you take off enough excess fluid to remain healthy. The nurse will check your weight and blood pressure on each visit, and will tell you if you have put on too much fluid since the last dialysis. It is uncomfortable for you if you have to have large amounts of fluid removed. You can feel faint and washed out afterwards, and dialysis sessions will need to be longer. Talk to your named nurse and work out how to manage your fluid intake.

Dietitian

Your relationship with the dietitian can be crucial to your long-term health. Once again, the key to the situation is to foster an equal and adult dialogue, with honesty and negotiation. If you try to conceal the times when you have not managed to follow your diet, you are only damaging yourself. Kidney patients have frequent blood tests, which can reveal their eating habits, so they have little chance of concealment in any case.

Renal social worker/counsellor

Most units have a renal social worker or patient counsellor, who may be able to visit you at home to discuss any issues that are concerning you. People often feel more free to be themselves when they are on their own territory, so the social worker can get a better impression of your circumstances on a home visit. The role of the renal social worker is to look at your situation as a whole, taking your illness into account, but focusing on your life *outside* the hospital. This may include your relationships, work, finances, and practical as well as emotional problems. If you wish, the social worker will communicate and liaise with hospital staff about your problems where this information may be useful. If you do not wish any information to be shared, confidentiality will be maintained.

If you need extra care at home, your social worker will be able to contact Social Services to arrange for an assessment of your needs. You may also want a referral to an occupational therapist, who deals with any aids and adaptations to your home, to make it easier to move around and manage daily living.

If your problems are concerned with your feelings, or relationships, support may be available from a renal counsellor. Not all units have counsellors available, but if you need help in coming to terms with difficult issues, ask for help. If your unit does not have a counsellor for kidney patients, ask your GP whether there is a counsellor attached to the GP practice.

Kidney doctors

Although most units strive for continuity of care, the reality is often much more complicated. You will not always be seen by your consultant (though you are likely to be under his or her care continuously). The more junior members of the team, the registrars, tend to be in post for shorter periods and, as the registrar is often the doctor you will see, you may find that you see many different ones over time. This can make you feel that your case has to be described all over again. Or, even worse, that the doctor has to spend the whole consultation reading your notes, or with eyes on the computer screen rather than on you. Unfortunately, there does not seem to be any way round this problem at present. Registrars may spend a six month or one year period in the renal unit, so you are unlikely to see the same person very often. Patients say that they have just built a relationship with one doctor when it is time for them to move on. A further problem arising from this lack of continuity, is that different doctors may give you different advice about your problems. This can be worrying for patients, but you need to remember that there may be several valid ways of approaching a problem. It does not mean that one piece of advice is necessarily 'right' and the other 'wrong'. Your doctor needs feedback and co-operation from you to decide, for example, which of many blood pressure tablets suits you best, or what dry weight you should aim for when dialysing (see the Glossary at the back of this book for an explanation of your 'dry weight').

Building a relationship with your kidney consultant

There has been a marked change in the doctor/patient relationship over the last two decades. Where doctors used to be figures of great authority, whose advice was followed as if infallible, they are now no longer regarded with unquestioning respect. Some, indeed, find themselves in a defensive position towards their patients, aware that their judgement will not always be accepted. In many ways, this less authoritative and unequal doctor/patient relationship is a great improvement. This is particularly true for people with chronic illness, where a realistic, long-term relationship is essential for the success of treatment. Much of the change has been due to a better informed public. Medicine has been de-mystified, not only by better communication between professionals and patients, but also by the media.

There are now many websites giving detailed medical information and advice. The Internet can be a very useful resource, but may also lead to problems in your relationship with your doctor. Patients sometimes ask about a new drug or treatment which they have seen mentioned on the Internet. This may be something that is worthy of consideration for you, but it may just as easily be something that is completely inappropriate in your circumstances. Sometimes patients read reports of experimental treatments whose usefulness has yet to be established. As their medical knowledge is necessarily limited, they may believe they are being denied the most up-to-date treatment, or that their request is being refused due to lack of resources.

The most important factors in your relationship with your kidney consultant (and indeed with every member of the team) are mutual respect and trust. This is not to say that you should give up all responsibility and follow advice blindly. You should feel able to discuss the reasons for a particular piece of advice, and receive honest answers to your concerns. But having sought the expertise of professionals about the management of your condition, it makes no sense to be constantly questioning their advice. If you cannot feel trust and confidence in your consultant, you should ask if you can be referred to another doctor since neither of you will be comfortable with the situation. No good doctor would be offended if you do this – they may even feel that you might be likely to get on better with a different consultant. After all, doctors are human too.

Clinic visits

Some people get very anxious about clinic visits.

> *I get very wound up before a clinic. A few days before, I start worrying. I suppose I wonder if there is going to be any bad news or any changes in treatment. I don't like uncertainty.*
>
> **George**

It is helpful, both for the doctor and for yourself, if you bring a list of your current tablets to the clinic. It is sometimes really hard to remember exactly what you are taking, especially during a short appointment when you are aware of time constraints.

Asking questions

When in doubt ask questions. If there is anything you are unhappy about, or unsure of, it is important you feel able to ask for clarification.

It can be useful to bring a list of things you need to discuss with the doctor. PD patients usually carry a small notebook with their daily weight and blood pressure record. It is sensible for all patients to make a note of anything they wish to report or ask. But remember that the appointment will probably have only 10 or 15 minutes allocated for it, so you may not be able to discuss more than two or three problems. If this will not be enough time to go through your concerns, ask your consultant for a longer appointment (say half an hour) on another occasion. Tell the doctor the most important thing first – for example, don't say 'I had terrible chest pains yesterday' as you leave the room.

Your doctor will be able to refer you to another member of the team if your concerns would be better addressed by a nurse specialist, dietitian, counsellor or social worker, who can provide advice and support.

Ask your doctor to forward a copy of the clinic letter (which he sends to your GP about a week after the appointment) to you. Many units do this routinely now. Keep these letters.

If the doctor you see at the clinic is not your consultant, make a note of his or her name.

The people you will meet outside hospital

General practitioners

Following referral to the kidney unit, you may not see your GP as often as before. Your consultant will keep your GP informed, by letter or telephone call, about your progress. You may continue to get prescriptions from your local surgery, except for the more complex drugs which you may need to collect from hospital. It is usual for GPs to suggest that you contact your kidney doctor if you have any problems, unless these are clearly unconnected with your kidney condition. Patients are sometimes sad to lose a close relationship with their GP, whom they may have known for years.

Home dialysis team

People who are on CAPD, APD or home haemodialysis have much less frequent contact with the hospital than those who attend for *hospital* haemodialysis. You will, however, be given the telephone number of your home dialysis team, who you can contact at any time if you are concerned. In many units (though unfortuntately, not everywhere in the UK at present) a member of the home dialysis team can visit you at home from time to time, to see that all is going well.

PD and other suppliers

You will receive a regular visit for delivery of your dialysis fluid and other necessary supplies. PD fluid is usually delivered once a month, although, if your storage space is very limited, you may get deliveries once a fortnight.

Helping the system

There are bound to be times when you get angry and frustrated by the way things happen, or don't happen, in the hospital.

Running a busy haemodialysis unit can be rather like running a production line, and at times patients can feel that they are a 'just another product', being processed. Nurses do not always have time to talk to you as much as they, and you, would like. Dialysis schedules may need to be changed unexpectedly from time to time. There may be delays in getting your treatment, often caused by hold-ups in transport, which have a knock-on effect in the unit.

Haemodialysis is like no other hospital procedure. It can mean thrice weekly contact with the staff, over four hours, for many years. You will probably spend more time with your dialysis team than with anybody else, excepting those you live with at home. They become your second family. Small wonder that there are good days and bad days. It is a credit to dialysis nurses that most patients are full of admiration for them and say that, in spite of being overworked and under pressure, 'the nurses are wonderful'.

There can be other frustrations. Appointments for non-urgent procedures may be cancelled and rescheduled. Minor problems can sometimes seem disproportionately large when one is coping with so much already. This is where it is valuable to be able to put yourself in other people's shoes; to realise that it could have been *your* emergency which caused somebody else's cancellation; to go with the flow, and be a little philosophical.

In a pressurised system, you can help staff by attending for appointments if you possibly can. Much time is wasted when patients forget (or decide not to turn up for) an appointment, without giving the hospital enough warning to enable somebody else to take their place. You can help by telephoning the hospital as soon as you know you cannot attend for a clinic or procedure.

Staff are usually doing their best, and much of the time everything runs smoothly, but, like so much in life, the system is not perfect. There are responsibilities on both sides.

Further information
Information about your rights as a patient can be found on the Patients' Association website (see page 141).

Most hospitals now have a PALS (Patient and Liaison Services) Manager who will be able to help you put your point of view across to the professionals if needed.

8
Work, leisure activities and holidays

Work makes me believe that life is normal – that I'm the same as everybody else. No one can see what is wrong with me. And those that do know, or find out, say it's hard to believe I'm on dialysis.

Frances

Some people assume that they will be unable to work on dialysis and give up their jobs shortly before treatment starts, but it need not be this way. There are both practical and psychological benefits in continuing work, and it is far easier to keep one's job than to get a new one following the start of treatment. So, continuing with your work can be a very important part of making a success of life on dialysis.

Practical benefits of work

Finances
One of the problems of illness is that it can hit your finances. Some employers keep you on full pay for a while, then reduce the money as time goes on. Others pay only the statutory amount, which is later paid by the Department of Work and Pensions. Those with a mortgage are most severely affected by a cut in their monthly income (see page 132).

Work is good for your health
People who give up work no longer have a reason for getting up and out of the house on a regular basis. Gradually, they may spend more and more time sitting watching daytime television, or more and more time in bed. They may lose interest in their personal appearance, where before they had taken a pride in looking smart. They take less and less exercise. As a result they lose fitness, feel weaker, and therefore spend even less time on activities. It is a vicious circle.

Psychological benefits of work

Maintaining self-image and self-esteem

As Frances says, work is part of your normal role in life. Your occupation gives you a role. You are not 'a kidney patient', you are a builder or gardener, a teacher or a school dinner lady, who happens to dialyse in their spare time. Paul, who has been a kidney patient for eighteen years, is a trained chef, but since the failure of his second transplant five years ago, he finds he does not have the energy to work full time.

> *When I first started back on dialysis this time, I spent a lot of time sitting around being sorry for myself. That's why I decided to go out and help people worse off than me. Everyone has skills they can use. The volunteer group asked what I'd like to do, and I chose the soup kitchen, because of my cookery training. I do two evenings at the weekend. The social side is really good too. You need to be doing something so that dialysis doesn't become your way of life.*
>
> **Paul**

Maintaining interests and contacts

At work, you have less time to dwell on your illness, because your mind is occupied with your job. You will also be out of the house and meeting others. This contributes to your sense of being just like other people, and reduces isolation and loneliness.

Keeping a positive attitude

If you are working, you are still a 'contributor' to the world. You are active rather than passive, so your sense of control over events is improved. You are a person who *does things* rather than a person who has things *done to* them.

Many people with kidney failure are in full-time work and, depending on their fitness level, may be able to undertake all but the most strenuous jobs. Obviously, those with a desk job are more likely to find work easy to manage, because no great physical exertion is needed. Dialysis patients have undertaken a great variety of employment, however, including manual work, production line or warehouse work and stock keeping, security work, printing, driving (including lorry driving), secretarial work, catering, teaching and nursing.

If you are working within the six-month period leading up to starting dialysis, there is every chance that you will be able to continue once your dialysis treatment is established. It is advisable to discuss the position with your Kidney Unit well in advance. Let them know that you hope to continue working, since this may affect the sort of treatment that is planned and the timing of the start of treatment. It also allows time for the unit to contact your employers with information about your likely ability to fulfil your previous commitments. This information cannot, of course, be given unless you request it. It may help very considerably in reassuring your employer.

Staff at the hospital will discuss with you how to fit treatment round your work. Some patients negotiate different hours, or a change of work within the same employment. Most employers are very helpful to kidney patients. However, they may, at first, be afraid that you will not be able to do your work properly. Others make it clear that the employee should seek other work.

One factor our contributors have in common is that they have no intention of letting dialysis become a way of life in itself. Those who were employed at the time of diagnosis have all continued to work, even if they are past retirement age. Those who were not employed carried on with everything they were doing before their treatment started. Some have desk jobs, but others do heavy physical work. Many have jobs that are physically, mentally and emotionally taxing.

It may be obvious that, if you have a chronic condition such as kidney failure, it is far easier to keep an existing job than to get a new one. There is a lot of ignorance and prejudice among employers, as the first three contributors demonstrate. All of these particular individuals decided that the answer was to go self-employed.

When I was first diagnosed, my employer at the market garden said he couldn't keep me on. They weren't thinking about me, they were thinking about their health and safety rules, and what would happen if I ended up under my fork lift truck one day.

So I decided I would go self-employed. My garden design customers are very good. I tell them about my kidney failure and they are amazed. They say 'you shouldn't even be standing up, you should be in hospital!' I enjoy showing them that I may have kidney failure but I've still got a life.

I was on CAPD then. Because my work is out in the field, on different landscape sites, I took my PD equipment with me in a clean box. I'd leave for the first site at 8.00 am, work at the first site, then do an exchange in the car and drive to the next site. It was a bind having to do the exchanges, but it only takes 20 minutes. Once I got adjusted to it and set up a regime, it came together very nicely. I was quite strict with myself at first, not lifting really heavy plant pots or paving slabs, or large sacks of compost. I started with smaller sacks, and worked up gradually. If it was a really heavy bale of moss peat, I'd get someone to move it on a sack-truck. You have to be careful and work out how to do things.

Chris

This was Chris's experience. There are many benefits in being self-employed, since you are able to arrange your work round your medical needs, clinic appointments, and the way you feel at any time. It is, however, important to keep up your contribution record and to pay a self-employed stamp. You will then qualify for incapacity benefit and a pension when you retire.

Andrew's experience shows how hard it can be to change jobs following the diagnosis of kidney failure.

I'm a builder. When I started dialysis I thought I'd get a part time job and re-train for something less heavy. I didn't think I'd be able to carry on with building work. I went to 40 interviews and when I said I had kidney failure, no one wanted to know, so I joined a friend (someone I was at school with), and went self employed as a general builder. The first three weeks were hard. I sometimes felt faint as if I was going to black-out, but my friend was very good. He said, 'just do what you can'. I was only paid for what I could do. I built it up gradually from there, and now I work full time and dialyse three evenings a week, on the twilight shift in hospital. I do bricklaying, stone laying, plastering – all the building jobs.

Andrew

I used to work for a computer firm. When I became ill, I had to take some time off (in fact I was in hospital several times). My employer said I was 'milking it', because I was off sick so often. That was when I decided to start my own company and become self-employed. My employer apologised when he found out how ill I'd been, but I'm happier being my own boss. If I need to take time off, I can.

George

Not all employers are unsympathetic. This is the experience of Rhys, a deputy headteacher and geography teacher at a boarding school:

I actually looked into early retirement when I was first ill. It was the uncertainty; I simply didn't know how I was going to respond when I was on treatment. I thought it sensible to consult the union official, who suggested using the Disability Act – employers have got to make allowances for you. That wasn't the sort of thing I wanted to use as leverage. My colleagues are all very caring – I've even had offers from colleagues to give me their kidneys. The school has been very good. I didn't have secretarial help before, but they provided that to make things easier. Lots of colleagues stepped in to help at first when things were difficult – it's the way we operate as an organisation. I haven't really had any problems with work – though I have cut down a bit. Instead of 70 hours a week, I do 60.

Rhys

Keith and Helen too, had sympathetic employers:

When things were not going well, I was falling asleep at work. I was working in a furniture factory then. They all knew about my condition, and when I would wake up an hour or so later they would act as if nothing had happened. They were very good. They told me to go to the sick room for a lie down if I felt too sleepy and to carry on when I could.

Keith

Diabetes caused my kidney failure, so I was on dialysis from the age of 25. I managed to carry on working part-time, but I used to get very tired. I worked in a supermarket. They were very good to me and let me work in the staff restaurant, so I could have a break when I needed it.

Helen

Very few employers will have already had experience of a person on dialysis. They may expect the illness and treatment to cause a lot of absenteeism, and create problems for other workers. They may, quite wrongly, think there is a risk of infection to others. Like Chris's employers, they may be concerned about health and safety issues. Since kidney failure is quite rare, it is not surprising that many employers don't know much about it and so make false assumptions. The truth, however, is that most kidney patients who continue to work after starting dialysis actually have better sickness records than their 'fit' colleagues. They are extremely keen to show that they can manage the job in spite of receiving regular treatment. It is a challenge. Where some people will take time off work for trivial reasons, many people with kidney failure won't take time off work unless they are very poorly indeed.

A letter from your consultant can make all the difference. It may explain that you should be able to do your job as well as anyone else – or, if the job is very heavy, make it clear what sort of work you could do.

I did have a problem with work because I was in the middle of changing jobs when I got my diagnosis. When I told my prospective employers that I had just been told I had kidney failure, they were not sure whether to keep the offer open. I needed letters of support from the hospital to explain that, once I had settled on treatment, there was no reason why I shouldn't do the job as well as anybody else. My employers know the situation, but I haven't told my colleagues about my kidney failure. I don't really feel I know them well enough yet. I don't want them to make allowances for me, or give me the easy jobs because I am not well, and they might do that if they knew.

Indira

Frances is past retirement age, and widowed. Her work not only helps with her finances, but keeps her in touch with old friends.

I work four days a week in the supermarket, on the checkout. I had to take a bit of time off to start dialysis. There was a chap at work in the bakery department who had had a transplant, and he said, 'There's really nothing to be frightened about. Come back to work when you have started dialysis.' So I saw the Personnel Manager and she said, 'If you're sure you want to carry on, fine. Just bring in a sick note for the time you need off'. I asked if I could cut my hours by one hour at lunchtime, to do my exchange, and she said that was OK. They were very good. They like to be kept informed. As long as they know where they are, they are happy to co-operate.

Frances

This is a very useful piece of advice. It is essential to keep your employer informed. If they don't know what is happening, they may think you are not going to be able to manage the job, and make you redundant. If you can explain that you will need a certain amount of time off to get established on your dialysis treatment, and then negotiate a staged or gentle return to work, you have a good chance of maintaining your employment. Important conversations should be backed up by a letter and, with your permission, your employers can talk to your hospital consultant.

Robert was lucky, because his employers already had a dialysis patient on the staff, and knew that it was possible to carry on normal work while being treated for kidney failure.

I work in London. I leave home at six in the morning – have done for twenty years. I'm now a project manager. I love my work, but I'd rather get home early, so I work from 7.00 am till 2.00 pm. They get their money's worth. When I get back, I work on my lap-top or PC, reading my e-mails and minuting the meetings I've been to in the mornings. I do a lot of that sort of work while I am on the haemodialysis machine. Since I got kidney failure, one of my colleagues has twice used my condition as an excuse for me when I have made a mistake. I don't appreciate that. I don't want to be treated as different, because, as far as the job goes, I'm not different.

Robert

Leisure activities

You might think that the effort of working as well as performing dialysis, would leave little time or energy for other activities, but you would think wrong. Do not give up any leisure activity without trying it first. It may be harder than before, but most activities are possible with the right support.

These are some of the things that our contributors fit into their lives, in addition to work and dialysis. Some people are fitter than others. Some have a huge amount of energy, some less, but all seem enthusiastic and engaged in life. There are people who lose interest in things once they can no longer participate as before. Not so Andrew or Robert, who are both interested in sport, and were active players. They now maintain their interest by helping the next generation.

I do a lot of walking. I also keep in touch with the rugby club I used to play for. I haven't the energy to play now, but after all I am over 40. I'm thinking of going back to training juniors.

Andrew

I get back early from work so as to spend more time with my kids. I have coached my son's football team every week since he was seven. He's 17 now, and I am still doing it. I don't run about anymore, because I get breathless, but I shout a lot! So that's Sundays taken care of. On Wednesday evening after I get off dialysis, I take my younger son training at the sports centre.

Robert

Paul also used to play a lot of football:

After going on dialysis I played in goal, which was less energetic. After my first transplant I gave up altogether, because in 'contact sports', you can get a hard blow in the tummy which can damage the kidney. Nowadays I go to the gym, but I admit I spend most of the time in the sauna. Very relaxing - – and I get rid of some fluid!

Paul

Self-development need not stop when you start on dialysis. These contributors took courses in subjects that were new to them:

I took a computer course last Summer. It will be useful in my job, but I did it mainly for interest.

Rhys

I enjoy swimming and walking. Also I decided to brush up my French – silly in a way, because I go on holiday to Spain every year, and can't use it. My daughter was taking evening classes in French and I'd always wanted to speak a foreign language well, so I went along with her.

Mary

At the volunteer group I work for, they organise courses and workshops. I'm doing photography, clerical training and a computer course – each one day a week.

Paul

Interest in other people and in helping them to fulfil their potential, was evident in a number of the contributors. Turning one's interest outwards, rather than dwelling on one's own position, seems to make for a positive attitude.

I take the school kids on field trips and visits – out and about all over the place. It was one of the hurdles I had to get over to get back to normality. The first one was a three day trip, with all the boxes and the machine. And I managed it. The last hurdle for me will be the school trip to Romania. I hope to do that this summer, then I can say that I'm really back to normal.

Rhys

I've got a passion for plants and also, of course, for people. I'm not just interested in getting myself well, but in helping others. I did the 'Timbo Run', for the BKPA [a leading kidney-patient charity], *raising money for kids on dialysis to have a holiday. It was a 24-hour drive around the country.*

Chris

At the soup kitchen we arrange outings both for the clients and for the staff. We take people on trips to the seaside – we've been to Brighton and Bournemouth – and we are going paintballing and bowling. We are helping other people, which can be stressful, so they organise loads of things for the staff. That's what you miss when you're not working – company and getting out and about.

Paul

Frances, like Mary, has had to learn to cope on her own after many years of married life. It can be hard to re-build one's life as a single person, and she admits it can be lonely, but with pets and a garden to look after she keeps active.

I hate the winter. I go to a couple of clubs in the evenings, but I don't get out that much, apart from walking the dogs. In the summer I'm always outside – gardening is one of my favourite hobbies, cutting the lawn and so on. I also like playing golf, though I'm not very good at it. I have played a few times since I started CAPD. And I love shopping. I lost my husband a year ago, and that changed the way I think about things. I have been on a real spending spree. We didn't have children, so there's nobody to leave the money to, so I decided to treat myself.

Frances

As Jenny and Indira found out, maintaining links with friends is an important part of normal life, which need not be lost if you start dialysis.

Six weekends a year, I go up to Lichfield. I go with friends on a self-development group for people working in textiles and it's very supportive. We all support each other. We stay in a B and B and we have a good laugh. I still do my art work and sewing. I don't work specifically for exhibitions any more. My husband and I like going out to eat with friends. We do a lot of that.

Jenny

I like reading, and visiting friends. I find it easier to spend time with friends than with my family or in-laws, who always treat me as if I'm ill and fuss about my diet. I don't like that, because I feel fine. If I have a day off work, I go with a friend and we drive to the next town for a day out, just something different to do. I went and stayed with a friend before Christmas, taking all my gear. People are so good, so interested. Once I had finished the overnight dialysis, the rest of the day was completely normal.

Indira

Reg remains a 'contributor' in every sense. Although on dialysis, aged 77, and living in a nursing home, he spends time looking after other residents and pursuing his hobbies.

I live in a nursing home since my wife died. I've been there five years now. I'm the only patient there who is self-caring. I do the gardening for the home, and bits of decorating. At the moment I'm pruning all the roses. Gardening was always my hobby. I help in the home, by pushing the other residents around in their wheelchairs, getting them cups of tea and so on. I did annoy the matron though. I dug up the turf of the back lawn to make a bed for my dahlias and chrysanthemums.

Reg

Whatever their age, these people are remaining active and engaged in life, both physically and mentally. Suffice it to say that many 'fit' people do a great deal less with their lives than these dialysis patients.

Driving

Kidney failure in itself does not affect your ability to drive. Some patients find that, at first, they feel a little unsteady immediately after haemodialysis. If this is the case, you should wait for a short while before driving home. This problem often disappears once you are settled on treatment.

If you have other physical problems as well as kidney failure, these may affect your driving. You should check with your doctor, who will have a list of conditions that should be reported to DVLC. It is also wise to check with your insurance company, to make sure you are covered. Anyone who has had an operation involving a general anaesthetic is advised not to drive for a couple of weeks.

Holidays

Patients sometimes fear that they will not be able to go away on holiday once they start dialysis. This is not true. Dialysis patients not only take holidays all over the UK, but also visit many countries all round the world, including Europe, Australia, India and Pakistan, the West Indies and the USA. A number of companies now run cruises, on ships which have their own dialysis unit.

If you are on haemodialysis it is necessary to make arrangements at a unit near where you will be staying. There are reciprocal agreements, covering the cost of treatment, between many countries, including those in the European Union. If you want to take a holiday in the United Kingdom, there are haemodialysis facilities at a number of holiday resorts, including some holiday camps such as Butlins. It is also possible to arrange holiday dialysis at some local hospital units, although many are too full to take visitors. Kidney Patient Associations, such as the BKPA, also run holiday units, and a number of private companies have opened small units for hospital dialysis near coastal resorts.

You can go almost anywhere you want for holidays, but bear in mind that some remote places will have few facilities for dealing with kidney failure, should you need to visit a hospital for any reason. Most of the world has well-developed kidney failure services and can be visited quite safely. Ask for advice at your unit well in advance of a holiday.

Travelling can be very easy for people on CAPD. Let your unit know where you want to go, and they will arrange for your dialysis supplies to be delivered to your holiday destination, whether in the UK or abroad. CAPD exchanges can be performed in airports and on aircraft flights if you plan a long trip. It may be possible for you to miss an exchange to make long distance travelling easier, but do discuss this with your PD nurse first.

Here are some of the comments on holidays made by our contributors.

Soon after starting APD, we rather foolishly booked a touring holiday round Scotland, staying at many different places. The first night we stopped, we were given a bedroom right at the top of a three storey house, and I had to haul the boxes and the machine up all the stairs. That was not a lot of fun. I learned then that it's better to think and plan ahead a bit.

Rhys

After my husband died, I decided to get out and about more. I bought a small carrying case for all my CAPD equipment, so I can take it anywhere.

I've visited my sister and my brother. One day I'll pluck up courage and drive to see my other sister in Bournemouth. I'm a coward when it comes to driving a long way in places I don't know. I haven't been on a proper holiday, but I'm not a holiday person. Never was.

Frances

Now I'm back on PD I often think, 'I wish we could just drop everything and go to Paris for the weekend'. It's funny, because all those years that we could have gone, I never thought about it or wanted to. When you can't, you suddenly wish you could. I know I could arrange it if I really wanted to — get the bags delivered to a hotel, and take the APD machine. It's quite portable. It's just that you have to be very deliberate and plan things in advance, rather than going on impulse.

Laura

Although she is in her seventies, Mary travels more than most people, going abroad several times a year. She usually goes with family or friends, and being Irish, likes to visit relatives in Ireland regularly.

I travel as much as I can. It needs planning — a lot of planning, when you are on haemodialysis. It's not easy but it's certainly possible. I even went to Canada to see relations. Getting to Spain last year, the phone calls to arrange everything cost the earth. I was trying to find a unit that would dialyse me free under the E111 form. In the end I went to a private unit, outside the Spanish health service, but they did accept the E111. They were extremely efficient, and they were in the town where I was staying. Otherwise I would have had to drive over an hour to Alicante. Once you've done it once, it gets a lot easier. I go to stay in Ireland every year, and I just write to the hospital and say how much I enjoyed the previous time, and they fit me in. I enjoy weekend breaks, because then you don't need to plan dialysis. I went to Prague for the weekend recently. It's a wonderful city, so much history and beautiful old buildings. I enjoyed that and will do it again.

Mary

Indira has family who are even further flung – and she would certainly agree with Mary about the need for planning.

I haven't been away yet, but I certainly hope to do so. The one thing that I resent is that the cheap late bookings are not practical any more, because you have to plan ahead. I did try to plan a holiday in Tunisia before

Christmas, but I seem to have chosen one of the only places that they won't deliver dialysis fluid! If I'd chosen Morocco it would have been fine. I'm sure we will go somewhere this year. I wanted to go to see my family in India, but I decided to wait until I had had a transplant.

Indira

People who have been dialysing for a long time – like Jenny – often have the confidence to take more adventurous holidays.

Because I do home haemodialysis with my husband helping me, I can use the portable Redy machine. We went to California two years ago for a wedding, taking the machine with us. After the wedding we toured round the United States. We had some pretty hair-raising experiences. We went on a cruise a year ago, all round the Mediterranean.

Jenny

Holidays can be difficult for older people, especially if they are widowed and have nobody to go away with. Many do not want to travel abroad, but holiday dialysis in the UK can be difficult to find. The Globaldialysis website gives useful information about where to find a dialysis unit abroad. Some older people with kidney failure need more information about what is available. They may find it helpful to have an arrangement within the unit, or more centrally. Being introduced to others who also want to go away, so that they may be able to have company on holiday can be very reassuring.

Further information

For more information on quality of life with kidney failure, see Chapter 7 of *Kidney Dialysis and Transplants: the 'at your fingertips' guide* by Andy Stein and Janet Wild, available from Class Publishing, London.

The Globaldialysis website (see page 140) gives information about dialysis units abroad.

9
Relationships with partners

My family say I suffer from mood swings. I disagree!

Rhys

Partnerships throughout the lifespan

Any chronic illness will have an impact on the family, and especially the partner, of the person affected. Research suggests that the support of those close to us, whether family or friends, is a very important factor that may affect our survival. Depending on the stage of life one has reached, partners and other close family members will be affected in different ways.

Young couples

Where kidney failure strikes a young person, the couple may have to put many plans on hold. This might include taking out a mortgage, moving to a different area for work, or (perhaps most important of all) having children. The person with kidney failure may feel guilty, that they are 'letting their partner down', and may doubt whether the relationship will last under such circumstances. Sadly, couples often don't talk about these feelings, which can lead to tension and distance in the relationship.

At the same time, the partner may also feel a great deal of anxiety, but try not to show it. Part of this worry can be due to not knowing enough about the illness. Lack of knowledge may make it difficult to judge what is a real cause for concern and what is trivial, as Chris explains:

She couldn't be a real support, because she didn't understand enough about things. If I was feeling ill and couldn't explain exactly how or why, she didn't know whether to give me a couple of paracetamol and tell me to get on with it, or rush me to the hospital. She was always so anxious about me, which didn't help me. But if I tried to shrug that off, she thought I didn't want her around. It all led to a breakdown in communication, and rows. She got quite depressed and felt let down.

Chris

It is very important for the partner to feel part of the team coping with the illness, and to gain as much knowledge as possible. This is why partners should be invited to pre-dialysis information groups. It is also a good thing if they attend clinic appointments with the patient, so that they can hear what the doctor says. Two sets of ears are better than one in any case, especially when the patient may have reduced ability to concentrate. It also helps the doctor to understand the home situation, and how much support the patient is getting at home.

It is very common for partners to say, 'He (or she) was complaining about so many things, and when he saw the doctor, nothing was mentioned at all. He told the doctor he was just fine. I really wanted him to *ask* about his problems, because I hear all about them at home, and I don't know whether there is anything that can or should be done'.

Many of the relationships are already under strain at the time of the diagnosis. It is not easy to be the partner of somebody with a long-term illness. If one shows a lot of concern, one is 'fussing'. But failing to show enough concern, or make allowances, mean one risks being seen as 'uncaring'. People who are facing the challenge of a condition such as kidney failure can become quite selfish and self-absorbed. And someone approaching the need for dialysis tends to be even less understanding towards others. They feel irritable, withdrawn and lacking in energy. This loss of enthusiasm for life often includes a loss of interest in making love to their partner. Some husbands and wives of patients have felt that they were no longer attractive or interesting to their spouse, not realising that this was just a symptom of the condition.

Middle aged couples
More mature couples can be in a better position, since they will probably have completed their family and will feel more secure in their relationship which will have had time to mature.

> *I don't think my illness has affected the family that much. My wife is a nurse and works from 6.00 pm until midnight, so with my evening dialysis we don't miss any time together. I wouldn't have home haemodialysis, because I think that would be an extra pressure on her.*
>
> **Robert**

Later life and bereavement
Older couples may both have health problems, so that the person with kidney failure (like Frances) may in fact be the fitter of the two, and have caring responsibilities for their frail partner.

We take things for granted don't we? I just assumed he'd always be there. Then he got lung cancer. At first he protected me by not telling me, but of course it became obvious. I remember him saying, 'This is all wrong, I thought it would be me nursing you'. I nursed him until two days before he died . . . In the end I couldn't cope with the care because I couldn't lift him.

Frances

Frances lost her husband two years ago, from cancer. Mary lost her husband from a heart attack. It is always a terrible thing to lose one's partner, but both of them expressed the feeling that it should have been they themselves who died. It was they who had the long-term illness, and they both expected to go first.

My husband supported me all the way. He used to do the shopping after dropping me off for dialysis, then join me in hospital for the last hour or two of treatment. We always played Scrabble, which passed the time. When he died suddenly from a heart attack, I was completely lost for a while. I was not only sad, I felt so angry with him for leaving me. I spoke to a bereavement counsellor who helped me a bit, but I still miss my husband all the time. I didn't expect to be the one left alone.

Mary

Sexual relationships

When a person with kidney failure is approaching the need for dialysis, a general lack of well-being often includes a loss of interest in making love. Partners in this situation are likely to feel that they are simply no longer attractive or interesting, or that their husband or wife has 'gone off' them. In fact, however, this decline in sexual interest is merely a common symptom of the condition. Couples sometimes find it hard to discuss the subject, and both parties may keep their worries to themselves.

Loss of desire

If you recognise this situation, you need to understand that this is not uncommon, and you are by no means alone. It is not anyone's fault, nor does it mean that there is necessarily anything wrong with your relationship. You should both be aware that the loss of interest (and, in many men, the inability to get an erection) is probably due to the illness.

Our sex life was affected because I totally lost interest, and she felt that it must be because she wasn't attractive to me anymore. She talked to our GP, who explained what can happen with kidney failure. I simply wasn't getting erections, and that knocked me for six! We stayed really cuddly, but I didn't like being touched sexually.

Chris

The problem may have a psychological basis, but it is more likely to have physical causes. Kidney patients may have hormone disturbances, which are a possible cause of sexual problems. Patients who are anaemic and lacking in vitality may not feel inclined to make love. This, combined with the other stresses of kidney failure, may affect your sex drive. In addition, some of the drugs given in renal failure can affect sexual performance. Do discuss this with your doctor.

Our love-life has definitely been affected. I can't get erections so easily, and the urge is not there so often. I'm not saying we don't make love. We do, but not so often, and it takes a bit longer.

Robert

Women with renal failure may lose any desire for sex, or may find it harder to reach orgasm. If dryness is a problem, there are many good products which help. Water based gels (such as Replens) are better than greasy ones such as petroleum jelly. You might also benefit from one of the hormone (oestrogen) creams, which are particularly useful after the menopause. Doctors and pharmacists can advise you.

Male partners are sometimes too considerate to suggest lovemaking, feeling that the woman would not be receptive due to her illness or might be harmed by intercourse. This can make her feel that she is no longer desirable, and lead to misunderstandings. Women with kidney failure may not have a strong libido, and may not reach a sexual climax, but they can still get pleasure from making love – and certainly from kissing and cuddling. One lady with kidney failure, when asked about her relationship with her active, healthy husband, told me that he was a great support, very good, very considerate, and never asked for sex. I suggested that she might like to thank him for his consideration by initiating lovemaking herself. She later said that it was a really helpful piece of advice because her husband had been thrilled to receive encouragement, and their relationship had got even better.

Maintaining contact

It is important for couples to try to maintain their affectionate relationship, even if full sexual relations are not possible. Touch is a very important sense which needs to be satisfied. Physical closeness and cuddling are comforting and maintain the bond between a couple. Most women who lose their sexual desire are still able to engage in intercourse, which helps to prevent their partner feeling rejected. However, partners should be patient and understanding if the woman is not as keen as she has been in the past.

Loss of the sexual side of the relationship is not often mentioned by carers, who may be embarrassed to talk about it. Or they may feel it is selfish to want sex when their loved one is coping with long-term illness. Joyce, who is now in her seventies, remembers the earlier years of her marriage. Her husband John has had diabetes for many years, and has recently reached the need for dialysis treatment.

When John first had diabetes, it was forty years ago. There was so little help for people then. Now there are even sex clinics – there was nothing like that for us. I just had to switch off sexually. But I missed it – I still do. Not everyone can switch off, so they find outlets outside, but I never felt like that. When you have finished putting someone to bed after working out what's been going wrong with them today, you don't think 'Now I'll dress myself up and go out to meet someone else'. You are glad to sit down and relax!

Joyce

People on peritoneal dialysis sometimes worry that sexual relations could be damaging, due to pressure on the abdomen, or dragging on the catheter. It is perfectly safe to have sex when on CAPD, or APD. If it is more comfortable, the position for intercourse can be changed to reduce pressure and minimise interference with the catheter.

Kidney patients are often restless sleepers, due to itching, restless legs or cramps at night. Some couples decide to sleep in different beds or even different rooms so that the partner can get a good night's sleep. While this is a possible solution, it may be better to tackle the cause of the problem by asking for advice. It can be sad for a couple to start sleeping separately. Both need the reassurance and comfort of closeness, especially if sexual contact is reduced due to the illness.

People on APD may find that the partner is disturbed by the noise of the machine during the night. Those who are light sleepers may find this a problem and decide that the best solution is to sleep in the next room. It is a very individual thing, which couples need to discuss frankly. Some couples, like Laura and her partner, do not find APD a problem:

Our love life hasn't been badly affected. We still sleep in a double bed. The APD machine doesn't keep my partner awake. It makes a gentle swishing noise, but he sleeps through it now. We make love either when I'm off or on the APD machine. My libido is quite low at present, but my partner is older than me, so it doesn't bother him. We make love once or twice a week. I have to say that if there was something to increase a woman's libido, I wouldn't mind taking it! I also think you can't put it all down to the illness. It could be tiredness or my hormones (they have put me on progesterone for heavy periods).

Laura

Male patients, who find it hard to get or maintain an erection, should discuss this with their doctor. There are several methods of overcoming the problem, one or other of which is likely to be suitable. Sildenafil (Viagra) and other drug treatments, are licensed for kidney patients and may be helpful. But Viagra should not be used by patients with heart problems, and this includes many dialysis patients. Other drugs are available now, which may be safer. There are also ways of producing and maintaining an erection without drugs, such as the vacuum device called an 'erecaid', which is safe and effective. Do not be afraid to ask for advice. There is nothing to be ashamed of in wanting a normal sex life.

If there are psychological reasons contributing to the problem, couples can ask to be referred to a trained psycho-sexual counsellor.

- **If you think that your sexual desire is affected by renal failure or your drugs, or if you think you would benefit from any counselling, please ask the nurses or doctors for advice.**

Not everyone is adversely affected. You may be one of the lucky ones who notice no difference in your desire or performance, or you may find that the start of dialysis helps you to regain your previous interest.

I have actually found that since going on dialysis, I have got my desire back. I feel so well now. For a year before I started treatment I really didn't feel like making love. I thought it was my age, or the menopause. But no, it's all come back and our lovemaking is back to normal.

Indira

Body image

Dissatisfaction with one's body can be one of the reasons for problems with lovemaking. If you lose the sense of being attractive, this is bound to affect your confidence. Usually, your partner is the person who will see you wearing the fewest clothes.

Unfortunately, everyone on dialysis has one or more operation scars, whether in the arm, to create a fistula, under the collarbone for a dialysis catheter or in the tummy for a Tenckhoff catheter for PD. The fistula can get quite large over time, standing out on the arm like a body builder's veins. Women with a well-developed fistula usually choose to wear long sleeves, which hides the vein completely. The dialysis line is invisible under normal clothing. The fact that others either accept or need not see your dialysis access, is no help if *you*, yourself, cannot accept it. Helen says that she didn't feel confident enough in her appearance, to work in a place where she met the general public:

> *I worked in the staff restaurant rather than on the checkouts at the supermarket because I was embarrassed by how I looked. I was often bloated and sometimes had a temporary neck line or a bandaged arm, or bruising from dialysis. I didn't want people to see me unless they knew me and understood.*
>
> **Helen**

Some people are more aware than others of the way they look, and worry more about any real or imagined blemish. It can be a great help if your partner accepts your access without any reservation.

> *I think my body has changed shape since starting PD. I think my legs are thinner and I've lost weight from my breasts, and my tummy is a bit bigger. But I'm not really concerned, because my boyfriend is not at all bothered by the tube for my dialysis. And if he's not bothered, nor am I. I wouldn't choose to go around in a bikini, but I would if there was a good reason. The way people are now, with all sorts of things dangling from their bodies, and piercings all over, I think it would hardly attract attention.*
>
> **Laura**

> *I was offered CAPD but I turned it down for cosmetic reasons. I just felt that I was young and still quite attractive, and my husband really fancied me, so I didn't want the catheter in my tummy. It was self-image. Now I'm*

older I don't mind so much. I would certainly consider it now, if my fistula stopped working.

Jenny

Helen was lucky in finding a partner who really understood and accepted her situation, because he too was a kidney patient:

After a couple of years on dialysis, I met Nick, who had just had a transplant. He was a great support to me and we later became partners. We helped and supported each other.

Helen

Keith feels that his CAPD catheter and the empty bag (which was not disconnected in the 1980s as it is now), affected his confidence and ability to make relationships with the opposite sex.

I felt like an old man with a colostomy. It was such a turn-off. At the age of 20 or 21, on CAPD, the thought of a relationship was ridiculous with that bag attached. I felt like a freak.

Keith

Luckily, modern systems do not involve having the bag attached between exchanges. It is quite possible that prospective partners would not have been put off, but if one *feels* unattractive, it is hard to engage in a relationship to put this to the test.

In discussions with partners, both male and female, very few over the years have expressed any negative feelings about dialysis access – whether for haemodialysis or PD. Most say that they love their husband or wife for themselves, and that changes to the body do not affect their feelings. It is hard, however, to convince some people who need dialysis access, that this is true. It is therefore their *own* acceptance of the catheter or fistula that is most important.

People on PD may notice some enlargement of the abdomen due to the two litres of fluid in the peritoneal cavity. Those with firm tummy muscles hardly show the fluid at all.

Of course, it can be more difficult if you are unmarried and looking for someone to share your life. Some single patients avoid contact with members of the opposite sex, because they lack the confidence to see themselves as desirable partners. They are also uncertain at what stage they should explain about their kidney failure.

Before I met my partner, I went out with several people. I told them about my kidney failure early on, because it is only fair to them. Kidney failure does mean there are restrictions, though I can get over most of them. There are ways of overcoming almost everything. The reason they need to know is that it can be very worrying to be with somebody who has an illness. There are times when it is upsetting, because it is not nice seeing somebody you love having a hard time. I told him, so he was prepared for that and knew what he was taking on.

Laura

It is very important for couples to maintain the physical closeness of their relationship, whether or not full intercourse is possible. Sometimes, the problem with a couple's love-making is due to a failure in communication. Some years ago, the wife of a patient came to me, desperate because they had not made love for two years. I spoke to the couple together. It transpired that the husband had occasional morning erections, but his wife, frustrated by their lack of contact, had resorted to sleeping pills at night. She was impossible to wake, let alone arouse, at 6.00 am. 'Why didn't you tell me?' she said. 'You never asked' he replied. Two weeks later there was a triumphant phone call to report success. If couples could only talk more to each other, most psycho-sexual counsellors would be redundant!

Fertility

Kidney failure causes many women to stop ovulating, and their periods become scant or disappear altogether. This inevitably affects their fertility. Very few babies are born to women on dialysis, and those that are, tend to be premature and need special care. Men also may find that their fertility is reduced.

My kidney failure affected our relationship because we wanted children. My partner is older than I am, so we wanted to start a family as soon as possible, but I was told that I had a low sperm count and that the sperm were not strong. The doctor said that we would have to wait until I had had a transplant.

Chris

The good news is that, after a successful transplant, most of these problems resolve. Many women with transplants have successful pregnancies.

However, you are likely to be advised to wait for a year or so after your transplant before trying to become pregnant. Some women are tempted to have a child as soon as possible after a transplant, whether they have the security and financial support of a long-term partner, or are facing parenthood on their own. This is very understandable – it may, after all, be the woman's only chance of having her own baby. The instinct to have a child is very strong, but lone parenthood can be difficult if the transplant fails, for example. The woman can then find herself trying to manage dialysis and motherhood on her own.

To have one's own child is a very strong and basic emotional need. Both men and women can feel inadequate if they are unable to have a child. Some couples choose to have artificial insemination from a donor if the man's fertility is low, but in this situation it is extremely important that the couple have a deep, understanding and loving relationship. It can be hard for a man to face the fact that the child is not his own, and that 'another man' was involved in the conception, however impersonally.

Further information

More information about positive living and sexual relationships in later life or chronic illness, see *Intimate Relations: Living and loving in later life*, by Dr Sarah Brewer. Available from Age Concern Books, London.

A helpful leaflet on *Sexual Relationships in Kidney Failure* is available from the National Kidney Federation.

The Relate website (see page 142) will give you useful links and information.

10
Carers, friends and the wider family

You have so little time for yourself, even to make yourself smart or do your hair. You don't think about yourself at all. My day is made up of what my husband needs. I get so exhausted. If there is a moment free, all I want to do is go and lie down for a while. And yet, in spite of this it is very rewarding. Every carer's story is different, yet in a way the problems are all the same.

Joyce

Partners as carers

Joyce is in her seventies, and has been looking after her husband John, who is diabetic, for many years. He is nearly blind, walks with great difficulty, and has just started dialysis. She has to do all his medication, because he cannot see to draw up his insulin. She also has to do all the correspondence, dealing with benefits and the taxman. John can no longer drive, so she ferries him to and from hospital appointments. It is no wonder she gets tired.

I never get an unbroken night. He goes to bed early, and when I go up he is just waking up again. He is very restless. I'd be better in a bed on my own, but he says that would be the end if we had to sleep apart after all this time. Sometimes I slip into the spare room to get a little rest. Nights are his worst time.

Joyce

Most patients put on a good face for hospital staff. But they can take out, or at least show, their feelings, frustration and worries with their nearest and dearest. Partners can find this very difficult.

If I get really fed up with things, it helps me to have a good cry. Afterwards I feel much better. The trouble is, it is difficult for those around me. I always say to my husband, 'Please don't get upset – I'm fine now'. But I know it distresses him. He can't let his feelings out as I can. He bottles things up. If he gets upset he sees everything I say as a criticism. He goes very quiet, and doesn't talk much. I've learned the pattern now, and don't try to get him out of the mood. I just have to leave him alone until he has worked through it himself.

Jenny

It is usually true that we are most 'ourselves' with those closest to us. They therefore see both the best and worst of us. The value of a good supportive relationship cannot be overestimated. As Indira found, support and love of a partner is one of the most necessary ingredients in coping well with a chronic illness.

My husband has taken most of the brunt of my illness. We are partners and I would have done the same for him if it was the other way round. He has been very patient. I don't think I would have been half as good a nurse to him as he has been to me. Our relationship has always been supportive, but it has become even more so. My husband has even offered me one of his kidneys.

Indira

The partner is often the one who ensures that tablets get taken when they should. This has already been shown from the quotes about drugs and medication. The diet, too, is often planned and organised by partners, especially when they are the ones responsible for shopping and cooking.

Caring for carers

Those who cope well with a chronic condition such as kidney failure, are seldom the easiest people to live with. They tend to be determined, even stubborn individuals who demand a lot of themselves and may also be impatient with others. But what about the carers? It may be a lot to ask that patients should think more about the feelings of those close to them, but if they are able to do so, they are storing up a great treasure in terms of support and happiness.

Many people whose partner or near relative is coping with long-term illness find it particularly hard to express (or even acknowledge) their own needs and feelings. This is all very well in the case of an acute illness, something short-lived. In the longer term, however, it can become extremely wearing.

Partners and carers need to have time for themselves, to recharge their batteries, although many find it hard to take such time, even if it is offered. Most feel guilty, although it is really important for them to get a break from the situation every now and then. There is help available if you need it. Relief carers can be arranged through Social Services, and respite care for a week or more is also possible. Few partners are willing to accept help, feeling that it is their duty to carry on alone. As a result they get overtired both physically, and mentally – like Joyce.

> *I have been offered respite care for him in a nursing or residential home, but I don't really want to get away. If I'm away from John I would be worried, all the time, that he was fretting. I'd feel guilty. By the time I came back, I know he would be in such a state because I'd been away and he couldn't see me. He'd feel guilty and so would I.*
>
> **Joyce**

Many partners live in a state of constant anxiety about the person they love.

> *I worry a lot. I'm a bag of nerves, I'm always looking and checking that things are not going wrong for him. I can't relax.*
>
> **Joyce**

Carers and partners find it very hard to express their needs, and often suffer in silence. Laura's partner was an exception. This quote shows how important it is to be able to communicate feelings in a relationship.

> *When I was in hospital for several weeks with a failing transplant, my partner was under a lot of strain. He was getting up at 5.00 am, working all day on a freezing cold building site, then driving 20 miles to visit me in hospital every evening until 9.00 pm. He then had to drive back home, eat and get to bed. My parents had moved in to stay, so they could visit during the day, and had taken over the house. He was feeling shut out and resentful. Luckily he told me how he was feeling, and that cleared the air a lot. We decided he should only come over twice a week. That gave him some time for himself. I was having such a lot of support from Mum and friends,*

but I knew that when everything had died down, he would be the one left at the end of the day.

Laura

Most carers feel isolated with their problems. Friends are sympathetic at first, but many drift away over time, feeling awkward in the face of long-term problems which are not improving. They may feel embarrassment, or simply not know what to say. A sensitive carer can be aware of this, and make matters worse by avoiding contact.

People don't understand. You may have a neighbour look in, but when they have gone all your problems are still there. I don't ask for help, because I don't want them thinking ' She's coming out of the house, let's not catch her eye in case she wants something'. So, I try to be independent. Anybody meeting me would think I was fine – they would have no idea what's going on in my head.

Joyce

When I asked Joyce what would help her, as a carer, she said:

You feel so alone. You feel there's nobody out there who understands, though I know that's not so. I need to feel there's somebody out there for me. There is a great deal for the patient, but little for the carer. Above all I need to talk and get it off my chest. I have friends, but they don't really want to hear it all, nor would I in their place.

If I had a bigger house, I'd like to invite lots of carers round for the evening, just to talk about their frustrations over a glass of wine. And then they could go back to the situation with some of the weight off their feelings.

Joyce

Joyce's situation is particularly difficult – partly because she has been having to deal with it for so long. The sooner you can become involved with support networks locally, the better. Most hospitals now have their own Kidney Patients' Associations. There are also national bodies such as the National Kidney Federation and Carers UK which will be able to provide support. The table opposite gives advice for carers and is adapted from the Kidney Patient Guide website for Carers, Partners and Friends.

Strategies for carers

- **Share the job**
  You may have got into the habit of believing 'it's your job and no-one else's' to support the person you care for. Look at how *you* can ask for support from others. This applies not just to the practical aspects of caring, but also to the 'job' of providing emotional support. You may find it helpful to suggest to the person you are supporting that they talk to someone else as well as to you – such as a counsellor – about their feelings. This may actually be better for both of you.

- **Don't try to 'solve' the unsolvable**
  Some carers feel it's up to them to find a solution when the person they are supporting is unhappy, angry or upset about their illness or its treatment. Actually, they may prefer it if you *don't* try to provide answers but just listen and understand so they don't feel so alone.

- **Don't overprotect the person you are supporting**
  You can actually do *too much* for someone. When this happens, not only are you likely to over-extend yourself, but the other person can feel powerless and dependent. This can leave them feeling even more frustrated with their illness.

- **Watch your stress levels**
  Taking regular exercise and learning relaxation or meditation can help to reduce stress and make you feel better able to cope with being a carer.

Feeling guilty

There is no doubt that living with the illness of someone you love can cause a state of chronic tension and tiredness. You may be giving up a lot of your time. You may not be able to do all you would have liked to do as a couple. You may have to take on tasks and roles that were previously your partner's responsibility. An outsider might see this as 'a burden', and feel sorry for you. But is this how partners themselves think? Of course they wish that the person they love did not have to suffer, or put up with a long-term illness. That goes without saying. But most say that, even if they had known what the future would hold, they would not have changed anything. This is sometimes hard for a person with kidney failure to believe.

I think my illness has taken its toll on my husband over the years. We do lots of things together, but I'm sure he wishes that he had a wife who could go on long bracing walks or even skiing holidays with him. I can't manage things like redecorating the house now, so an awful lot falls on him. I think he lives with the constant fear that something will happen to me. If I go into a really deep sleep at night, he wakes me up because he is afraid I have died.

Jenny

If couples can discuss matters openly, it often transpires that the partner is aware of insights and benefits from the situation. Laura and her partner have been through a lot together, financial struggles adding to their worries about her kidney failure. She used to run a sandwich bar but has now retrained as an aromatherapist, while her partner is a struggling builder.

My partner says that he doesn't feel my illness is a burden to him. It helps him to put his own problems, like his business, in perspective. He says it has shown him what is important, and made him grateful for his own health and the fact that we are together. We have been quite poor with his business struggling, and my business struggling. But we are not poor in our heads. We like each other's company and don't go out much.

Laura

Sometimes the partner's anxiety is expressed in overprotection, which can prevent the patient achieving all that is possible.

My husband became more protective, in fact too protective when I was first diagnosed. He treated me like an invalid. He'd say, 'You're doing too much', but I knew my limitations and I didn't feel like a piece of fragile china. He became less anxious as time went on and once I started dialysing he encouraged me to do more. He didn't let me use my kidney failure as an excuse for not doing things. That was a great help. He was a wonderful support.

Frances

Many people with kidney failure feel that they are a burden to their partners and, if they are older, to their children and grandchildren. It can help to balance up the situation if, like Mary, they are able to give something back.

I do a lot of baby sitting for my grandchildren – I'm in demand for that sort of thing. It's something I can do to help. That was the worst thing about giving up my work as a midwife – I didn't feel needed anymore. We all need to be needed.

Mary

Some people, like Rhys, can also find it hard to accept help, if they have been the 'strong' one who gave to others in the past.

In my job at the school I am trying to 'give' all the time. It's a difficult exercise to turn the tables and say I'm going to be receiving help from others now. I find it very hard to be the recipient of other people's concern.

Rhys

Attitudes of parents and the wider family

When a patient is widowed, children and grandchildren often take over the caring responsibilities.

I'm lucky with my children and grandchildren. That's been a great factor in helping me to carry on. They can sometimes be overprotective. This New Year I wanted to be on my own after losing my husband, because we always went out together. Two of my daughters were having a party, and wanted me to come over, but I had to pretend I was going somewhere else because I knew they would worry about me.

Mary

Being protective

I was 19 when I started dialysis. I lived at home with my parents who were naturally very anxious and protective. I reacted very badly to the whole thing. For the first year or 18 months I was looking for somebody to blame for what had happened and I made everyone's life a misery.

Keith

It can be very hard for the parents of young adults who develop kidney failure. Their reaction is often to become over anxious and over involved with treatment, refusing to acknowledge that the patient is grown up and should be taking responsibility for themselves. This can be particularly difficult for young unmarried adults, on the brink of making their own way in the world. Suddenly their childhood and dependency seems to be prolonged. Parents no longer want them to move out of the family home, fearing that they will not look after themselves properly.

My parents want to wrap me up in cotton wool. They won't let me take responsibility for my own illness, even though I lived away from home for years.They fuss over me all the time.

Chris

Paul lived with his mother when he started dialysis, but later moved into his own council flat. His mother seems to have understood his need for independence:

My Mum has been OK about it. A lot of my family have moved back to Jamaica, but she lives close by. She is always there if I need her and would do things for me if I wanted, but she has encouraged me to be independent. I've got into a routine with housework and laundry now, and don't need her help. I talk to her on the phone twice a week, so she doesn't worry about me.

Paul

In some cases parents are unable to come to terms with the illness. They often feel guilty because they are unable to 'put things right' when their child is suffering in some way. They ask themselves whether they have done something wrong, or whether they could have prevented the illness.

My mother simply can't deal with it at all. That's been one of the worst things about it for me –the hardest thing to cope with. I try to tell her about it, but it either seems to be over her head, or she had her own opinions about it. She has not been a support to us, because she cannot accept what has happened to me.

George

Many parents of kidney patients feel terrible at the thought that their children may die before them, particularly if their own age or state of health means they are unable to donate a kidney for transplant.

Following transplantation, the long 'adolescence' of the young kidney patient can finally end:

My relationship with my parents is good now. I have my own house, I'm independent and not so much of a worry to them. My Mum has done enough worrying. I didn't leave home until after my second transplant, when I was in my mid-thirties.

Keith

Cultural differences in attitude to illness

In Asian culture there is a rather different attitude to illness from that found in the West. There is great reticence in admitting to illnesses and disabilities, which are kept quiet. This can create problems within families.

My mother has not even told her sisters, or any of my cousins in India about my illness. In my culture, if you have a disability, you are somehow only 'half a person'. One does not speak about it. It is not perfect, not pure, to have something wrong with you. It is part of our religion to be healthy and normal. You do not flaunt it if you are not 'whole' as a person. At the end of your life you are meant to die in a 'perfect' state, taking everything that you were given, back to God, as it was meant to be. I am cross with my mother about this, because it makes things so difficult. I am really worried about visiting India, because my family have no idea that this has happened.

I feel that people who do know about my kidney failure 'accommodate' me and my illness, when they have no need to do that. I don't need to be accommodated, because I'm alright.

Indira

This reticence about discussing illness makes it even more important for Asian patients, especially women, to have a support network involving other people with the same problem, with whom they can freely communicate. Their difficulty, according to Indira is 'finding each other'.

I met an Asian optometrist, a medically trained man, who asked me about my kidney failure and the drugs. I was surprised by his interest and knowledge about things, and said so, but he explained that he had worked in a hospital. It took him another half an hour of conversation with me before he admitted, almost reluctantly, that he himself had had kidney failure and was a transplant patient. Why could he not tell me at once? He said he hadn't told anybody at work. I then asked if he knew another Asian patient I had met at the unit, and at that moment somebody walked into the room, and he said that he did, but he quickly changed to speaking in our language to keep it private. It all had to be 'hush hush'.

Indira

Effects on children in the family

Children are remarkably resilient. Those who grow up in a family where a parent has a chronic illness usually accept the whole situation without question. Trouble seems to arise when parents feel guilty about what has happened. They may worry that children have been deprived in some way due to the illness, and overcompensate – usually with material things. What children need most is their parents' love and attention. Both of these may be hard to supply when you are absorbed in your illness and short of time. Some patients, like George or Indira, say that they have changed their priorities and realised what is most important in life following the onset of kidney failure.

Since I've been ill, I've adapted my life so that I have more time with my children. I used to think about work all the time, but my outlook on life has really changed. I come in for treatment at 8.30 pm, so that I can be with them until they go to bed. I take them out every weekend – nothing special, we go for walks and to the park. We do far more together than we did before I was ill.

George

I have tried to cushion them from my illness a bit. It's not fair on them, because it's my disability and I don't want it to affect them. Of course they realised that I was very unwell, but, by going back to work as soon as I could, I tried to keep things normal. They do jobs for me like carrying heavy things upstairs.

Indira

Many patients comment on the fact that their children are more thoughtful, responsible and caring than average, due to growing up with a parent who needed their help and consideration.

I think, when I started dialysis, it made a huge difference to me to have young children to look after. It was such a motivation to carry on as normally as possible. I do feel that my kidney failure has had a tremendous effect on them. It must have been very difficult for them when they were little, with me in and out of hospital. They both developed bad stammers. My son used to help with my home dialysis from the age of eleven. They were never wild teenagers. I feel they missed out on that. They were so responsible and thoughtful.

Jenny

Older children are often more anxious than young ones. They have not 'grown up' with the illness, and find it harder to accept.

My daughter is away at college at present, and she feels marginalised. She keeps ringing up wanting to know about my condition all the time, and likes to be told of any changes. My son, deep down, is worried about me and cares – a lot. He'd like to go round the world, but won't because he wants to be close at hand if something happens.

Rhys

Children are experts in picking up 'atmospheres'. Even very young children seem to be aware if parents are worried or distressed. They may feel even more puzzled and insecure if parents try to conceal that anything is wrong. As George says, it is usually best to be honest and open.

My kids are four and eight years old. They know all about my illness. I've explained it all to them. They come along to my hospital appointments. That was a decision we made early on. My wife's father had cancer and it was always kept quiet, you couldn't mention it at all. She learned from that. It's better for the kids to know all about it, rather than imagine things worse than they are.

George

Some people find there are positive effects on themselves and their families. This was Robert's experience and that of Indira's family.

We have decided to make Tuesday night our 'family night'. We all do something together, which didn't often happen before I was ill. My 17-year-old always wanted to go out on his own. Sometimes we stay in and have a meal, or we all go out for a pizza. It could be anything, but we do something as a family and it's made us closer.

Robert

I think it's made our family closer. I don't argue with my Mum so much. Everything's more chilled out, more relaxed. Maybe it was me being all 'teenager'. I was being selfish, but now I'm more aware. I used to get angry with Mum and argue, but now I'm more laid back. I make allowances for her. I don't let a lot of things bother me anymore 'cos I realise they're not important. This has shown me what's important. I was very worried about Mum before the diagnosis, so it was a relief to know what was wrong –

because there was something that could be done about it. I still worry, but not so much. It is always in the back of your mind though. I'm more like my Dad. He just quietly gets on with things.

Indira's daughter, aged 17

Even young children are quite able to help parents, or grandparents with their treatment. Children who feel involved and useful rather than excluded from the realities of what is happening, are less likely to be worried by dialysis, since it ceases to be a mystery.

For more information

Information about kidney disease and specific advice to carers can be found on the website (see page 141).

The charity, Carers UK, will also provide information and support (see page 139).

For a refreshing look at life from the carer's point of view – and how to survive it, see *The Selfish Pig's Guide to Caring* (see page 137 for details).

The author's wife suffered from Huntingdon's disease, very different from kidney failure, but carers in all situations often find they have much in common.

11
Lifestyle for kidney patients

Living *well* with kidney failure should also enable you to live *long* with it. This is as much your own responsibility (if not more so) as it is the responsibility of the medical and nursing team. To a great extent, you can control your own health and prolong your life.

Kidney patients who consistently 'break all the rules' not only live less long, they also feel dreadful. Living well with kidney failure is living with sense and self-discipline. But as our contributors show, it does not have to mean living without enjoyment.

Positive health measures

Those people who are treated by dialysis for kidney failure seldom die as a direct result of their illness or treatment. The most common cause of death in kidney patients is the same as for the general population – heart attacks and strokes. Kidney patients have a slightly greater risk of heart disease than normal, due to problems with high blood pressure, and a tendency to a high cholesterol. However, there are are a number of things you can do to minimise the risks of heart disease.

Smoking
It is well known that smoking causes lung cancer. It also carries a risk of damaging blood vessels and making a heart attack or stroke more likely. So, whether you have kidney failure or not (but particularly if you do) you are increasing your risk of an early death if you smoke. If you want to live long and you smoke, of course it makes sense to give up. But this may not be as easy as it sounds. Ask your doctor for help if you feel you need it. You are likely to find the medical profession today helpful and sympathetic, as it is now widely understood that tobacco is addictive and giving up can be very hard. However, there are good nicotine replacements available which may help you. Some people also find hypnotism helpful, while others find acupuncture more effective. Your doctor may be able to refer you for recognised therapies such as these – it would be worth asking.

Exercise
Most of our contributors mention some sort of exercise among their leisure activities. Some had previously been very active, but following their kidney failure they adapted to gentler exercise.

> *I like going for walks, getting out into the countryside. I'm not as fit as I'd like to be. I used to go jogging quite regularly, and I don't feel up to that yet. I walk two or three miles. Sometimes I do that both morning and evening.*
>
> **Rhys**

Many patients with a chronic illness such as kidney failure, feel that they are 'frail' and should avoid doing things that they used to enjoy. This is not true and can be damaging to both physical and mental wellbeing. It is easy to get into a vicious circle. If you do less, you become less fit and lose muscle strength. This makes you feel weaker, so you do even less. This is a depressing way to live, and can make you feel you are an 'invalid' when there is no need to be one.

Your general health will benefit from regular exercise. This does not have to be vigorous. Work to your limits and make a point of being as active as you can. This will keep your muscle strength up, and help keep your heart, circulation and bones strong. It will also encourage you to feel good about yourself, positive and interested in life.

Exercise will depend on your age and what you like to do. Some younger dialysis patients enjoy skiing, rowing and other very active sports. One Wiltshire patient even ran a marathon while on PD! Exercise does not have to be so strenuous. Contributors have mentioned swimming, gardening, golf, walking the dog – or even going round the shops – as ways of using the joints and muscles to keep you fit and interested in life. Dancing – including ballroom dancing, line dancing and salsa – are excellent exercise, and have been mentioned by patients along with the more 'serious-minded' visits to the gym. For those who get breathless on exertion, yoga and pilates, which are based more on stretching than aerobic exercise, are particularly suitable.

Fluid and diet: following the guidelines
The importance of diet and fluid balance to kidney patients cannot be overstated, as this quote shows:

> *When we went on the dialysis cruise, we dialysed every other day in a unit on the ship, which was German owned and run. Most of the*

passengers were German. That was a real eye-opener. The dialysis staff asked me how long I had been on dialysis, and when I told them, 22 years, they were amazed. They said that the German dialysis patients didn't usually live as long as that, and when I asked why, they said 'because they have no self-discipline'. I couldn't help seeing what those patients were doing. They were putting on 4 or 5 kilos of fluid between treatments, and I noticed they were eating piles of chips and everything they shouldn't have. I would rather feel better and live longer, but I suppose it's their choice!

Jenny

Keeping to diet and fluid recommendations are at the core of living a long and enjoyable life with kidney failure. All the excess fluid that you take in between treatments must be removed by dialysis. If you are on haemodialysis and have gained 5 kilos in fluid weight, it is a shock to your system to have that amount removed rapidly. It can make you feel faint and cause your blood pressure to drop suddenly. The extra fluid in your system puts a strain on your heart, causing it to become enlarged and damaging the heart muscle itself. A lot of extra fluid may also make you breathless, because your lungs become waterlogged.

Haemodialysis is much more comfortable if the amount of fluid to be removed is only one or two kilograms. Your blood pressure keeps stable and you feel better afterwards. Dialysis needs to be a gentle process, putting as little strain on your body as possible. It cannot be gentle if you need to take huge amounts of fluid away in a 3- or 4-hour treatment session.

As discussed in Chapter 3, the diet need not be a great trial. You can balance it and 'negotiate' the things you would really like to eat, like George:

If I have a bit more potassium today, I balance it out. If I want to have a glass of wine today, I cut out the mushrooms tomorrow. We have a lot of fresh fruit and keep the fats low. It's helped us to feed our kids a healthy diet, healthier than most kids. We all eat the same food. I don't eat differently from the family.

George

Fluid restrictions can be harder to tolerate.

The more I am told not to drink, the thirstier I feel. I know when I have drunk too much because I don't feel so well, and get breathless. I'm getting better at keeping to the limit as time goes on, but it's hard in hot weather.

Indira

I tend to have small cups, or half cups where I used to have a full one. I always have some idea of how much I have drunk during the day. You find you are keeping a tally without even thinking about it.

Laura

Some people find it hard to give up drinking large quantities of beer. It is of course, not the alchohol that is damaging, but the quantity of fluid. There is nothing wrong with having one or two 'shorts' during a visit to the pub. Neither gin nor whisky is high in potassium though, unfortunately, *wine* is. Most people find that they can 'negotiate' their potassium intake, so as to enjoy a glass of wine with a special meal.

Tea can be taken in moderation, but instant coffee is quite high in potassium and should be avoided most of the time. Freshly ground coffee has less potassium, and can be drunk occasionally – especially if, like Jenny, you choose it instead of another high potassium food. In hot weather, some people find it better to suck ice cubes (which are cooling, and last quite a long time for a small amount of fluid intake) or chew gum, instead of having a cold drink.

Fasting

Fasting is an important practice in many religions – the best known being the obligation for Muslims to fast during daylight hours during Ramadan. Certain categories of people are excused fasting, and this would apply to anyone on dialysis. However, some devout Muslims do like to try to fast during Ramadan despite health problems, if they possibly can. If this applies to you, do talk to your doctor – as well as your religious leader – about the safest and most appropriate way to approach this.

Understanding your medication

Whether you are on dialysis or have had a transplant, your medication will be very important. Understanding what you should be taking, and why, will help you to feel in control and increase your motivation. There are a few general points that apply to all kidney patients – being aware of these may make your drug regime easier to cope with:

- Know what your drugs are for (and how they work) as this will help motivate you to take them. Know the dosages too.

- Some drugs are long term and prevent complications arising at some time in the future – this may make benefits in the short term difficult to appreciate. (As an example, blood pressure tablets lower your longer term risk of strokes and heart attacks.)

- Take a complete list of your tablets to every appointment with the doctor.

- Arrange a meeting with a renal pharmacist to go through the tablets on this list.

- Tell your kidney consultant or registrar about any new tablets (for any condition at all) prescribed by your GP. (This is for several reasons: some drugs can mix badly with other drugs in unexpected ways; some drugs would normally be removed from the body via the kidneys – so you may need a different dose from someone with healthy kidneys – and some have the potential to speed up kidney damage.)

- For the same reasons, you should not take any over-the-counter or herbal medicines without first asking your kidney consultant.

- If you have had a transplant, don't let *anyone* change your tablets except your kidney registrar or consultant. This is very important.

Blood pressure and cholesterol
Keeping a normal blood pressure helps to protect your heart and arteries. If you have been prescribed blood pressure tablets, it is important to carry on taking them. If you think they are having side effects that are inconvenient or unpleasant, discuss this with your doctor who may be able to prescribe you an alternative. There are literally dozens of different blood pressure tablets which all act in different ways, so there is a good chance of finding one that suits you.

You may also be given a 'statin' to lower your cholesterol, since a high level of cholesterol in the blood risks 'furring up' the arteries.

Phosphate and calcium
Many of our contributors found it hard to remember to take their phosphate binders. These are tablets – such as Calcichew, Phosex, Alucaps or Renagel – which reduce phosphate levels in the blood. They are needed to

prevent too much phosphate from being absorbed from the food you eat.Too much phosphate causes weakening of the bones. It is sensible to keep them on the table where you eat, so that you are less likely to forget them. They can be rather large and difficult to take, but if you can do so regularly, your bones will be in far better condition as time goes on.

Immunosuppressant drugs following transplant

If you receive a transplant – from either a dead or a living donor – you will be prescribed a regime of immunosuppressant drugs to help prevent your body from 'rejecting' the kidney. The most commonly used immunosuppressants are:

- **Ciclosporin** The most important drug used to prevent rejection of the new kidney. Unfortunately, if the levels of ciclosporin in the blood are not monitored very carefully, it can damage your new kidney and stop it from working ('ciclosporin toxicity'). There can be other unpleasant side effects such as gum damage and excessive hair growth. A drug called **tacrolimus** is now being prescribed as an alternative, but this can also have severe side effects including an increased incidence of diabetes. Both drugs have been associated with an increased likelihood of developing a form of cancer called lymphoma.

- **Azathioprine** Another drug to suppress the immune system, which is used in combination with ciclosporin/tacrolimus and a steroid. This reduces the production of red blood cells, so a likely side effect is anaemia. It can also cause liver damage. Mycophenolate mofetil is now being used as an alternative, but this too can cause anaemia.

- **Prednisolone** This is a steroid drug and can therefore cause thinning of the skin and easy bruising, as well as swelling of the face (giving the 'moon face' traditionally associated with steroid taking). It can also cause diabetes, and in some patients can weaken joints and bones.

Cautions if you are taking immunosuppressant medication

If you have had a transplant, the importance of taking your immunosuppressant tablets *cannot* be overstressed. One missed dose could cause your body to start rejecting the new kidney and cause the transplant to fail. The side effects may be difficult to deal with, and you need to talk to your doctor about this. It is in the interests of your medical team to give your new kidney the best possible chance of working, and this includes doing everything they can to help you feel comfortable on your drug regime. If a particular drug is really upsetting you, it may well be possible for your doctor to prescribe you an alternative, so ask – and keep asking. Your doctors won't know how bad you feel unless you tell them.

Most immunosuppressant medication will be prescribed in large doses at first, but these will be gradually reduced as the new kidney becomes stable in your body. This is likely to mean that side effects will reduce too.

While you are on immunosuppressants, you will be more prone to infections than before. Any infections you do catch will be likely to hit you harder than before as your body's natural defence mechanisms are subdued by the drugs. So you will need to take even minor infections very seriously, and report them to your doctor straight away.

Immunosuppressant medication also increases the likelihood of developing diabetes, anaemia, and certain types of cancer including skin cancer. You will therefore have to be particularly careful to eat a good, balanced diet, and whenever possible to stay out of the sun. Don't sunbathe, and if you do have to go out of doors in strong sunlight, wear a hat and a high factor sunscreen.

Many other drugs react badly if you take them with immunosuppressant medication. So don't take any other tablets, for anything else, unless you have first cleared their use with your kidney consultant. You should also avoid grapefruit and grapefruit juice, and alternative or complementary preparations such as St John's wort and echinacea.

To protect the transplanted kidney, Helen not only takes her immunosuppressant tablets, but takes great care with her diabetes:

I used to run very high blood sugars. That was what caused my own kidneys to fail. Once you have a new kidney, you really look after yourself, so I'm very careful with my sugar levels. They have been more stable since my transplant in any case, but I'm determined not to damage my kidney by letting them get too high.

Helen

Being in control

Remember that all the aspects covered in this chapter are things which are under your control, and they all have an influence on how well, and even how long, you live. Take responsibility for your own health. You are in the best position to know what is good for you and what isn't. Your body will tell you when you are going wrong.

> *The most important thing I have learned is to go by the rules. I started by trying to cut corners with my PD. I was getting slap-dash about things and that didn't work. It resulted in a peritonitis infection. Later I went onto haemodialysis. At first I wanted to skimp treatment, by decreasing my dialysis time. Finally I accepted that I felt better on the full four hours, and it was better for my health.*
>
> **Chris**

Most people find that structure and routine help them to follow their treatment with least effort. Jenny is no exception to this.

> *On home haemo, I could change my dialysis days whenever I want, but I'm reluctant to do that. I feel that self-discipline and routine hold the whole thing together. Of course, I will change the day for something really special, but in the normal way I like to keep the structure going.*
>
> **Jenny**

12
Ways of coping

Once I had the catheter in for PD, I thought – well, I've got to accept it and get on with it. Accepting it was definitely the key to moving on.

Frances

You may have formed some impressions of the way our contributors cope with their illness. They are very different people, with very different lifestyles, but they have certain things in common. These are a few of the topics that were mentioned by several (and in some cases by all) of them.

Acceptance

'Acceptance' seems to be the starting point for many people. If you cannot accept what has happened, you are, in a sense, emotionally stuck. You may be full of bitterness and resentment. You may be looking for something or somebody to blame for what has happened. All your energies, which should be used to cope with your situation, are wasted on thoughts which cannot change anything.

The biggest thing is acceptance. Once you have accepted that you are 'a renal patient', you are halfway there. A lot of people waste time saying 'What have I done to deserve this?'

Chris

Acceptance can take time. It varies a great deal from one person (and from one situation) to another.

From my own experience, you need to give yourself time and be aware that you go through phases of mental acceptance. You can't accept it all at once. At first it seems like the end of your life, but it isn't. Life can be lived and enjoyed with kidney failure. Once you have come to terms with it, you can move forward.

Rhys

There seems to be a process, or journey towards acceptance, which is hardly ever smooth. There may be setbacks, when you think you are back at square one, but then there is a leap forward. It is a bit like the old game of snakes and ladders, but in the end you reach your goal. Acceptance is easier if you have known for some time that dialysis would be necessary. If the diagnosis is late, it can take longer for you to come to terms. Shortly before she received the telephone call for her transplant operation, Indira said this:

> *I do still feel resentful, because if I had been diagnosed earlier, I might have had a transplant by now. Some people go on the transplant waiting list even before they start dialysis. I needed time to adjust to the fact that I'm unwell, and to tackle problems one at a time. I never had that chance, and I feel angry. I know I'm lucky and that I have had a marvellous service from the NHS, but it doesn't stop me feeling resentful that it's happened, and happened in the way it did.*
>
> *Indira*

Denial

> *I think I must be in denial. All my friends say, 'It's all right! If you are tired, or not well, you can say so', and I say, 'No, I'm feeling well'. Perhaps I'm in complete denial!*
>
> *Indira*

It has become very fashionable to talk about people being 'in denial'. This is seen as the opposite of acceptance, yet a degree of denial can be a useful way of coping with a difficult situation.

The truth is, that unless most of us were 'in denial' most of the time, the world would be a very boring place indeed. We all ask each other, 'How are you?', almost automatically, and equally automatically, we reply, 'I'm fine'. It would cause real surprise, not to mention irritation, if we answered truthfully, listing exactly what minor problems we were currently suffering from, every time we were asked. Yet if people with kidney disease say they feel well, their friends will not accept this reply, and automatically assume the person must be in denial.

So what does this phrase – 'in denial' – really mean? Not facing up to things? Unable to see the reality of the situation? Knowing the truth at an intellectual level, but refusing to acknowledge it at an emotional level? Any, or all of these things?

In order to describe yourself as 'in denial', you have to have recognised the reality of your position, the thing that you are denying. What you really mean is that you know the truth of the situation and have chosen to ignore, or make light of, your problems because you find it easier to cope that way.

Some people, including kidney unit staff, say that a person is 'in denial', when they mean that they are not sticking to their fluid restrictions or diet – in other words, they are not taking advice or caring for themselves as they should. This is a rather different problem.

One of the contributors claims that he 'does not think of himself as a kidney patient' and is therefore 'in denial'. Yet he attends regularly for dialysis, driving himself 20 miles in each direction, after a heavy day's work, to do so. Provided you are willing to act as if you were a kidney patient, following most of the advice you are given most of the time, and attending for treatment, it really does not matter whether you define yourself as a kidney patient or not. In fact, almost all our contributors say they do not think of themselves as 'kidney patients'. Rather, they define themselves in terms of their jobs, their families, their interests and their beliefs.

When I go home after dialysis, I stop being a kidney patient.

Robert

I suppose I'm in denial, but it's working very well for me!

Andrew

Being in control

Taking an active part in treatment
The great majority of contributors stressed the importance of being actively involved in their treatment. All seemed to believe that they could influence their health for the better. Rather than feeling at the mercy of fate or luck, they felt that they were, to a great extent, in control of the situation. 'Patients' are often seen as passive recipients of treatment, controlled by the medical and nursing profession, but our contributors all demonstrated an active attitude towards both the professionals and their illness. Several stated that gaining information was the key to taking control.

Find out all you can, so that you don't get scared and you feel you have some sort of control over things. Ask what is happening, check things out. Then you feel you are a person with an active part in the process, instead of just a patient being treated.

George

I think you need to ask as many questions as possible, and get knowledge and understanding about the illness. That helps with acceptance, and also I feel in charge of my treatment. I am going to 'manage' my kidney failure.

Chris

Life is very precious. You have to make the most of it. How I get on, is really down to me. The staff do all they can, but it's up to me to control what happens.

Jenny

The next two comments highlight the co-operative relationship which can and should be developed with renal unit staff:

It is a shared responsibility. I bow to the expertise of the doctors and nurses, but they can only put in the ingredients. It's down to me to determine how treatment goes.

Rhys

The dialysis nurses are great. I listen to them and they listen to me. They let me experiment with my treatment according to how I feel. For example, I asked if I could take off less fluid for a few treatments, to see if that would affect the amont of urine I still pass. If it doesn't work I'll go back to taking off more fluid.

Robert

In psychological terms, all of the above can be said to have an *internal locus of control*, which is a characteristic often found in people who make a success of projects they undertake. Those who have an *external locus of control* feel that they have little influence over what happens to them. This makes them feel helpless, especially in the face of illness. Once you know that you can make a difference, you are no longer helpless.

Having outside interests

> *It took a lot of planning, but I stayed focused on my work. A lot of people I dialysed with could only focus on being a kidney patient, and they made themselves really miserable.*
>
> **Chris**

Without exception, the contributors to this book had outside interests and enthusiasms, whether connected with their work, family or hobbies. They all continued to pursue these interests after starting dialysis. Some had to modify what they did, to find ways round their limitations, but they did not give up the things that interested them.

Flexibility – 'going with the flow'

Any condition that extends over many years, will have ups and downs. Frustrations, such as cancelled appointments, problems with transport to hospital and changes in haemodialysis schedules, can all contribute towards the downs. Individually, they may be relatively minor things, but for someone who is already putting up with an exacting treatmen regime, these irritations can sometimes seem to be the last straw. As a kidney patient, it will pay you to learn to shrug off such problems if you possibly can, rather than letting them make you angry. You need your energy for more important things. There are many ways of managing frustration, some of which are mentioned by our contributors in the next section.

> *I think I've learned to be quite laid back. I have had some cancelled appointments, like when I went to see the transplant surgeon, but it's always for a good reason. It's not as if they do it on purpose to annoy me! Another person was probably in greater need of the surgeon at the time. One day it could be me.*
>
> **George**

> *I feel very sad for nurses and doctors who get flak from people when there are hitches.I reckon you spend more energy being negative than being positive, so you should be using that energy to pull you through, not for fighting the system.*
>
> **Rhys**

Both these responses demonstrate an important way of converting negative feelings into positive ones. This is to consider things from someone else's point of view. The ability to put oneself in another person's shoes is a valuable and helpful trick.

There may be more serious problems from time to time. Many hospital visits are due to problems with dialysis access (fistulas, Tesio lines or dialysis catheters) resulting in short admissions for 'revisions' to be done. Haemodialysis cannot work well if the access does not provide a good rate of blood flow to the machine. The fistula may need to be moved from the wrist to the elbow, or created in the other arm.

After several years on dialysis, some kidney patients may need to have their parathyroid glands (four pea-sized glands in the neck) removed to protect bone strength. Patients sometimes feel they have put up with enough procedures over the years and resist having this operation. It can, however, be an essential factor in avoiding softening of the bones (which can lead to fractures).

Life on dialysis can never be fully predictable, which makes it all the more important to be flexible in the face of setbacks.

> *I'm very flexible. I go with the flow. I believe that you have to try to be really happy inside yourself, rather than depending on outside things to make you happy. If you are happy from within, whatever happens, wherever life takes you, you are still the same person.*
>
> **Laura**

Finding positive aspects

Most of the people who have contributed mentioned positive things that had resulted from their illness.

> *I wouldn't change anything. I wouldn't have the priorities I have now if it had not been for my illness. I have realised what is important.*
>
> **George**

> *I see my kidney failure as an opportunity – a challenge. How you deal with it is the important thing. Just occasionally, I use it as a good excuse not to do something.*
>
> **Rhys**

> *My illness has made me appreciate and value life a lot more. I don't take things for granted now. I think every day should be enjoyed.*
>
> **Laura**

It is easy to blame dialysis for any and every limitation, but one can find ways of adjusting the way one sees things:

> *Sometimes I think I'd like to be able to go away on impulse, and I can't because of taking the machine and fluids. But my partner bought me a dog for my birthday, knowing that I wouldn't be able to travel so much now. That was clever of him. Now I can tell myself it isn't because of dialysis, it's because I'd have to find a dog sitter. My dog is one of the good things to come out of my treatment . . . she means so much to me.*
>
> **Laura**

Setting goals and planning for the future

> *There's lots of things I still want to do and I can't see any reason why I shouldn't be able to do them.*
>
> **Rhys**

Many people with kidney failure say that they see little point in making future plans. This is usually because they see their condition as unpredictable. Some have, perhaps, booked a holiday and had to cancel due to an unexpected complication or admission to hospital. Rather than be disappointed again, they decide that it is not worth trying to do anything adventurous. This is an example of a 'self-imposed' limitation. If you have no plans, it is true that you cannot have your plans ruined. It also means that you are denying yourself the chance of doing something you would enjoy. Chris and Jenny have both learned to live in the present.

> *At the start it's best to take it a month at a time, then start to set goals, maybe planning a year ahead. I have got several plans. This year I want to do a bungee jump and I'd like to go hot air ballooning. I am also planning to go skiing. My real ambition is to see the South American rain forest. I don't know how to arrange that yet, but I will get there somehow!*
>
> **Chris**

> *I don't look too far forward, and I never look back. I do plan things to look forward to, because I need goals. I plan what I would like to be doing a year ahead, but I don't think, 'What will my health be like in a year's time?' You just can't tell. We are planning to go on another dialysis cruise at present.*
>
> **Jenny**

Laura creates her happiness by appreciating the here and now. She loves her work, and her dog, and the life she has created at home with her partner. She does not spend time wishing for unattainable things.

People say you must have hopes and dreams. I don't think I do, because I'm happy with my life as it is. It may not be perfect, but it's good.

Laura

It is quite possible to combine living a day at a time, with having future plans. The mind is quite capable of running two 'programmes' at the same time:

You can't know the future, but at least you can shape it a bit. I try to live both day to day, making the most of things as they are, and planning for the future. My future is getting my business into shape. I want to adapt my work so as to spend more time with my family.

George

I'm actually very happy in the here and now, so I don't plan ahead much. Every day should be enjoyed. I have tried to make my 'present' ideal rather than looking to the future. Having said that, my partner wants us to move to Scotland, and I'm considering that. I would also love to get a place in Spain, convert a ruin or something.

Laura

Having goals can even be a way of prolonging one's life. A very frail elderly lady on dialysis was in hospital, and not expected to survive. She told members of staff that she was determined to live to celebrate her golden wedding. This was a year away. In spite of having numerous illnesses, she achieved her goal, dying a week after the date she had set. Others have kept going to see a great grandchild born, or to receive a visit from a relative living on the other side of the world. It is amazing how much influence we have over our own lives provided we have something to aim for, something to live for.

Involvement with patient associations

Some people want to involve themselves with other kidney patients or with projects connected with the illness, while others want to distance themselves from everything to do with kidney failure.

As I don't see myself as a kidney patient, I don't want to get involved in the Kidney Patients' Association. A nurse asked me if I'd like to join, but I said that I don't want to be reminded that I'm different. I want to lead my life in the normal world.

Frances

I really enjoy meeting others in the same position as me. I go to most of the meetings of our Patients' Association. I think it's a great source of support, and a way of helping other people. We meet in each other's houses and if anyone is lonely or has a problem we can always ring each other up.

Mary

At my last unit, I was a Patient Representative. We tried to make things better for people on dialysis. The unit needed a dishwasher, so we got half the money from our Patient Association and raised the other half ourselves. We also got televisions with videos supplied for people dialysing. We met the consultants once a month to express views on behalf of patients.

Chris

I get involved with the pre-dialysis information groups. I know what it felt like to be a new patient, and I want to be able to tell them that it's not the end of the world.

Rhys

Those on PD or home haemodialysis visit the hospital rarely, so can begin to feel that they are the only people in the world with kidney failure. There are benefits in meeting other patients occasionally, as Jenny discovered:

I hadn't realised how much the dietary advice had changed over the years, nor had I learned about the overnight peritoneal dialysis machine, which is a comparatively new treatment. That's something that I might consider one day, if my fistula ever packs up.

Jenny

A lot of people also get support from the Internet in chat rooms. The Kidneywise website has a popular one, as does Kidney Patient Guide (see page 123). For patients who may be nervous about using a chat room, the National Kidney Federation offers a message board service which enables patients to leave and answer messages posted there by other patients. This service – called Talkline – can be found at www.kidney.org.uk

Feeling fortunate

A number of contributors volunteered the opinion that they were lucky, or fortunate in some way.

In a lot of respects I feel I am lucky, because kidney failure has changed my attitude to life for the better. I'm better off than a lot of people.

George

I'm so grateful to be alive now. I heard about a man who needed dialysis forty years ago, as a young man. There was no routine treatment in the UK at that time. He had to go to America and then to Canada to receive treatment, working his way to pay for dialysis. I could do without kidney failure, but yes, I do think of myself as fortunate.

Rhys

I feel very lucky that I live in England. In India, where I was born, the treatment is not so available or so advanced. I have spoken to friends in India and they say, 'You're in the best place'. I know I'm lucky, but I suppose still feel resentful that it happened at all.

Indira

I don't exactly feel fortunate that this happened, but I do think that I have the strength and optimism to get myself better.

Chris

I think I am a fortunate person. I have such a loving family; also good friends, not many but close. I couldn't have managed all these years on dialysis on my own.

Jenny

Being positive about dialysis

Taking on dialysis should be as positive as joining a regular fitness course at the gym, or getting a really important part time job. Yet many people see it in negative terms. They see the things they might not be able to do. They see lots of rules about diet and fluid. They see limitations. Almost grudgingly, they allow themselves to be put on dialysis, because there is no other option. But they resent the treatment and all that goes with it.

They are not *dialysing*, they are *being dialysed*.

Starting treatment should feel like the most positive decision you have ever made. If you want to live, you should really want to dialyse, and if you want to live well, you should want to dialyse well.

Yes, I am positive, but there's not anything very special or unusual in that. In most things I'm an optimist, but of course I sometimes have pessimistic thoughts – we all do, especially when we're ill. Some of the patients really live around dialysis. They can be pretty negative.

Mary

My biggest personal achievement has been to become positive. I used to think that I couldn't do things because I was a kidney patient, but I've surprised myself. I used to be a rather pessimistic person, but dialysis has changed me. I think I have much more focus, and inner strength.

Chris

I'm sure it helps if you are positive. Being negative actually affects your immune system. They did an experiment with actors, making some play positive roles and others negative ones. At the end they measured their immune response and compared it with previous levels. Those playing positive roles had increased their immunity and the negative ones had dropped.

Laura

It really is a matter of choice. When you have a chronic illness, you may feel that choices have been taken away from you, but the most important one remains. This is whether to close in upon yourself, shrink your horizons and concentrate on your illness – or, on the other hand, to open yourself to all that is still possible and explore life to the full.

For more information

A number of websites (including the website of the National Kidney Federation, the Kidneywise website and the Kidney Patient Guide) offer information and advice, and provide chat rooms. See Appendix 3 for more details.

13
What helps when you hit low points?

You may have gained the impression that the contributors have had an easy time, but this is far from true. Three have had failed transplants. One has had to change from PD to haemodialysis due to bouts of peritonitis. One was not diagnosed until the last minute, and is still struggling to reach acceptance. One is beginning to suffer the complications of long-term kidney failure, and two have lost their husbands since starting treatment. One nursed his wife until her death and now lives in a nursing home. They have all had low points.

When asked how they coped with periods of depression, there were many different responses, but one reaction was shared by all of them: 'There are always people worse off than me.'

When I have low points, it is my wife and children that pull me through. I am so lucky to have them and they mean everything to me. They motivate me to carry on.

George

In bad moments I comfort myself with music. For me, music is like an antiseptic which heals the hurt. It's like the sun coming out and making you open up like a flower. I use techniques like that to lift my spirits when I get depressed.

Chris

I do like to have a good cry. I find it really helps me to release tension. I also make myself imagine a worse scenario, because that's always possible, and then be thankful that things are not as bad as they might have been. That's my self-preservation mechanism. When I feel really low, I just let it happen. You may need to feel low for a while. It's the mind's way of having a rest and regenerating. You'll come back out of it – you always do.

Jenny

I still get weepy bouts over my husband's death. Everybody has low patches. I just have a good cry. Another thing I do is to have a long bath. I sometimes stay a couple of hours in the bath, which is one of my ways of relaxing. Sometimes I fall asleep and wake up when the water starts going up my nose, or gets too cold! I'm a great source of mirth to my kids. They tease me something rotten.

Mary

I just think that there's lots of people worse off than I am.

Frances

The place of faith, belief systems and spirituality

It is difficult to live life to the full without having or developing a sense of purpose and direction.

Whether one has a firm religious conviction, or doubts about the existence of anything beyond ourselves, most human beings need to give meaning to their lives, and especially to suffering. All those who say, 'What have I done to deserve this?' have, at the very least, a sense that life should follow some sort of rules. If you are good, you should be rewarded. If you are bad, you should be punished. The thought that life is totally random and accidental goes against our deepest instincts and needs. Yet it is painfully obvious that bad things can happen to good people.

Those who cope well with something as 'unfair' as kidney failure, might be expected to have some religious belief to help them through bad patches and give them strength. One of the contributors does, indeed, have a deeply held faith, but most are agnostic (hopeful, but unsure). Some found their faith re-kindled. Some had no faith at all.

I used to be more religious, but I think it made me feel that I must have done something bad to be in this situation. Years ago when I started dialysis, we had a lovely minister who was very involved in the Church School where my children went. He gave me a tremendous amount of support when I had my transplant. I went through a very bad time, thinking that I had benefited from someone's death. He showed me that you can't think like that. At the moment, I'm feeling more and more against organised religion, because of the political side of it – wars and things.

I have been on Yoga and meditation courses which I have found a great help. I meditate before every dialysis.

Jenny

I am Roman Catholic and go to church twice a week. Most times, when I'm positive, I feel that there is an afterlife, but there are times when I doubt it. Sometimes I wonder if there really is a God at all, but I continue with my religion. It gives me a sort of framework.

Mary

I'm quite spiritual, but not religious in the ordinary sense. I go through phases. I just try to be a good person and have a positive effect on other people. That's why I do the massage for the sick and terminally ill. I like to think there's an afterlife and that there's some kind of God. I have this funny feeling that He's probably speaking to me every day, and I'm not recognising it. I wish I had absolute faith.

Laura

I am a Christian, and it's the core factor in all I do. I have had work colleagues and children in the school saying to me, 'But you are a Christian, so why has this happened to you?' You don't 'buy into' God as an insurance policy. You can't say that, because you are a good person, you are exempt from things like illness. So that's a non-issue. I don't blame God for what happens. I do my best to honour Him whatever happens to me. I couldn't do the job I'm doing, let alone cope with the illness, without my faith in Christ.

Rhys

I was brought up in the Hindu tradition. I didn't think I had a religious faith, until this happened. It's almost as if I need there to be somebody up there for me to lean on. I started to believe, because it could have been worse, I could have died. I feel there is a power up there. It isn't that it can change anything, but it helps me feel stronger. I must be getting my strength from somewhere.

Indira

I'm not religious, but I think I have spiritual awareness. For me it is definitely music that puts me in touch with things outside myself, and helps me through bad times.

Chris

These contributors all had a religion – or at least a sense of something spiritual outside themselves. This obviously helped them, but faith is not essential to cope well with life. George, Robert and Paul were different:

I was brought up as a Catholic, but I am not religious at all now.

George

No, I'm not religious at all.

Robert

What do I do when I hit a low patch? Well, I like a smoke if you understand. That helps me chill out. I'm not religious, though I was brought up a Catholic, and it is a church group that organises the Soup Kitchen. But, no, religion isn't for me.

Paul

Alternative and complementary therapies

You have to be careful with alternative remedies. St John's wort and echinacea for example. They may be good for people with normal kidneys, but can be dangerous for us. So I'm a bit wary. Some Chinese remedies may be bad too. If there are any supplements that I think might help, I ask about them. I saw a psychic healer once. It was expensive and I just kept getting worse, so he said it must be 'karmic' – fate. You do have to be careful.

Laura

There is an important difference between 'alternative' and 'complementary' therapies. Alternative treatments are taken *instead* of those prescribed by orthodox medicine, while complementary therapies run alongside and support them. In the case of complete kidney failure, there is no option to treat with an 'alternative' to replace dialysis treatment, since none exists. Some complementary treatments may, however, help people to feel better. Laura herself provides complementary therapy in the form of massage, Reiki and aromatherapy.

Problems can arise with some, though by no means all, complementary treatments, due to the fact that no particular training, qualification or licence is required to set up in practice. This can mean that you are being treated by someone who hasn't been properly trained, so always ask about their qualifications. Reputable practitioners will always be happy to confirm their background and training.

Homeopathy, acupuncture and chiropractic are all recognised and in some cases performed in NHS hospitals. If you consult an osteopath or chiropractor for back, neck or other joint pains, it is important that they are aware that you are a kidney patient. Manipulation needs to take into account the state of your bones.

The treatments that should always be discussed with your doctor are those which involve taking medicines and dietary supplements. Herbal and 'health food' remedies can contain powerful substances which may be unusually toxic to kidney patients. This may be because healthy kidneys are necessary to remove them from the body, or because they contain unacceptably high levels of potassium.

The usual reason for seeking complementary therapies is to find ways of helping you as a 'whole person', rather than treating your medical condition alone. It is quite easy to forget or neglect the rest of you – mind, body and spirit – when so much energy is put into treating one aspect of you, your kidney failure. Since they deal with you 'as a whole' these therapies are sometimes called 'holistic'. Many involve the senses, such as touch and smell, which can have a calming and healing influence on the mind and body. Our feelings can be powerfully and positively influenced through the senses. Anything that makes you feel better and more positive – such as relaxation, meditation, music, reflexology, massage or the use of essential oils – will help you to put things in perspective. You may also find you have more energy for coping with your problems.

Most of our contributors agreed that relaxation was very important to them, though they had varied ways of helping them to release tension. Anger and frustration seem to be a part of everyone's life nowadays, but especially so for those affected by chronic illness. These negative feelings sap one's energy to deal with problems of everyday living. Kidney patients, more than most people, need to conserve and direct their energy in a positive way. Holistic and complementary therapies – such as yoga, meditation, visualisation and Reiki massage – can help you to let go of negative feelings. You may then find the calm centre of yourself. The same is true of religious and spiritual experience. All are methods of spiritual renewal through emotional release, leading to a peaceful and positive state.

Further information

More information about the range of complementary therapies available, and how they might be able to help you cope better with the situation you find yourself in, see *Know Your Complementary Therapies*, by Eileen Inge Herzberg. Available from Age Concern Books, London.

The British Complementary Medicine Association (BCMA) publishes the *BCMA National Practitioner Register*, listing practitioners who belong to member organisations.

14
Living well

For my first seven years on dialysis, I was never once asked how I felt about it all and how it was affecting the family – until one day I lost my temper. I cleared the doctor's desk for him – and got sent to a psychiatrist. I went in to see the psychiatrist and said 'I don't know why I'm here, I'm not mad you know', and he said 'No, you are a perfectly normal person, trying to deal with a very abnormal situation'. That was a wonderful way of putting it.

Jenny

Jenny's 23 years on dialysis cover half the history of dialysis itself. There have been great medical advances during this time, but human beings and their needs have not changed. Sadly, the psychological care of those facing the 'abnormal situation' of relying on dialysis, has not advanced as dramatically as their physical care. In an overstretched Health Service, it is natural for limited resources to be concentrated on the medical needs of patients. Yet one could ask 'what is the point of keeping people alive, without doing everything possible to make that life worthwhile?'

Even strong and determined people, like Jenny, need support from time to time. Counselling is available in some units, and may be very helpful. One cannot (and should not) always expect psychological support from the family, since they are too closely involved. Also, one does not wish to upset them by unloading one's natural frustration and anger. Where counselling or psychological support services are needed but lacking, kidney patients and their families should not be afraid to say so. They should call their kidney unit's attention to their needs, without fear of being thought weak or 'mentally unbalanced'. They are, indeed, normal people in abnormal circumstances. And many of them, like our contributors, can triumph over their difficulties and lead rewarding lives.

Living well and positively does not mean that you have to maintain a mask of cheerfulness all the time. There are times when you may need to feel low for a while, and, as Jenny says, give yourself time to recover and regenerate. A full life is not the same as an 'easy life'.

'Living well' means surely experiencing both good and bad things, without losing your positive outlook, or your interest in what is going on around you, or your sensitivity to others. Above all it is the ability to feel both happiness and sadness, rather than shutting the door on your feelings. One of the possible reactions to long-term illness can be a sort of indifference – a 'hardening of one's shell'. At first, this can be a protective measure, but finally a prison in itself. All of our contributors seem to be open to their feelings. They are connected to life through their interest in all aspects of life and in other people.

Their advice to others with kidney failure is remarkably consistent, depite their great differences in age, personality and circumstances. Here are their 'top ten tips':

1. Don't panic – life goes on! Make the most of it.

2. Try to accept what has happened. Maybe not all at once, but bit by bit. Then 'go for it' wholeheartedly. Discover ways that kidney failure can be a good thing in your life.

3. Ask questions. At your own pace, find out all you can about the illness and its treatment.

4. Take an active attitude to treatment as early as you can, to gain a sense of control. Use all the unit staff to your advantage.

5. Communicate with your doctors and nurses in an adult and equal relationship. Follow most of the advice you are given, most of the time. (Perfection is not possible.)

6. Continue with work, hobbies, holidays and other activities if at all possible.

7. Make realistic plans, as goals and rewards for yourself, and enjoy achieving them.

8. Go with the flow when there are setbacks, and keep going.

9. Don't be afraid to ask for help when you need it.

10. Dialyse to *live*, not just to stay alive.

It is appropriate to give the contributors the last words in this book.

Laura is a great example of dialysing to live. Here is her description of the day on which I interviewed her:

Today I got up; drove to do a home massage for a client; came back; picked up a friend and took him to the supermarket; came back; did another massage for a client; dropped my friend off with his shopping; took all my cardboard (mostly empty PD fluid boxes) for recycling; came home; dusted and cleaned the bedroom; set up my dialysis for tonight; changed the sheets; vacuumed downstairs; watched Neighbours; then I have two more clients for massage and aromatherapy later this afternoon. Then I shall go out and walk the dog, then get supper for my partner, then watch TV, then bed and on to my APD machine. That's how my days are. I hardly ever sit down!

Laura

This is a normal busy day for a housewife running a business, yet Laura, whose transplant failed four months ago, fits PD into her usual schedule.

Chris set up his own landscape gardening business, after a very difficult start. He wants you to know that, even if it takes time, anyone can come to terms with dialysis and lead a worthwhile life.

When I started haemodialysis I talked to a lot of other patients. Many of them seemed knocked for six by what had happened to them, but I believe that everybody can find a way through it. Some will take three weeks, others may take three years. It took me a number of months before I could say I had a positive and balanced attitude to the illness and treatment.

Chris

Rhys meditated on the difference between those people who allow the illness to rule their lives and those who live well:

Part of it is whether you see yourself as a winner, or a loser, a person with influence, or a victim. If you spend time thinking that life has dealt you a bad hand, it just makes your outlook even worse. All difficulties and tragedies either strengthen or weaken you as a character. What happens to you, either draws you towards the positive side or the negative. That applies to everything in life, as I keep explaining to the children at the school. The important thing is that 'You have the choice'.

Rhys

Appendix 1
Information on finances
for renal patients

Insurance and mortgages

You will need to declare your kidney failure for most life and insurance policies that you may want to take out. Policies you have taken out before developing kidney failure may not be affected, but if you are in any doubt you should check with your insurer at the earliest opportunity.

Providing you are generally fit apart from kidney failure, you should be able to get a mortgage. The Kidney Patients' Association (National Kidney Federation, see page 141) has details of brokers who can find 'kidney friendly' insurance companies, so contact them if you have any problems. See Appendix 3 for the address.

Just occasionally, there is an unexpected benefit. Some 'Critical Illness' Insurance Policies include kidney failure in the conditions for which they will pay off your mortgage in full. Do check the small print.

Employment rights and sick pay

Even if you intend to continue with your employment, there is likely to be a period towards the start of dialysis treatment when you are unable to carry on working. If you are an employee with a contract entitling you to full pay for a certain period, followed by half pay for a further period, you may well be able to get back to work before suffering financially. If you are self-employed, however, or entitled only to Statutory Sick Pay, you may find your financial position is badly affected. The best way to ensure that you do not lose out on any benefits available to you, is to visit a Welfare Rights Agency or a Citizen's Advice Bureau. The rules and conditions on benefits change frequently, so it is best to consult someone who is up to date with any new legislation. The following information is no more than a guide, suggesting which benefits you may be able to claim.

Free prescriptions

You may already get free prescriptions, because you receive Income Support, are over retirement age or are on a low income (apply on Form AG1). Those who have certain conditions such as diabetes are also entitled to free prescriptions. If you are a kidney patient, you are entitled to free prescriptions from the time that you have access formed for dialysis. This may be a fistula, a dialysis catheter or a Tenckhoff catheter for PD treatment. If you have not yet got dialysis access, you cannot claim free prescriptions, but would probably benefit from a pre-payment card.

DWP benefits

Incapacity Benefit

- In order to get Incapacity Benefit, you need to have paid National Insurance Contributions.

If you are working, and need to come into hospital, remember to ask the ward nurse for a certificate (sick note) to send to your employer. If you are unemployed, the sick note should be sent to your local benefit office. If you are not fit for work when discharged from hospital, you will also need an outpatient sick note, which you can get from your GP. Once you have been on Incapacity Benefit or statutory sick pay (from your employer) for 28 weeks running, you may have to be assessed by the Department of Health who will decide whether you are incapable of all work (rather than unable to do your usual job). Certain people will not have to take this test and will automatically be allowed long-term incapacity benefit. Those who are exempt from the test are:

- those who are registered blind;

- those who have severe heart or lung problems leading to very reduced exercise tolerance;

- those with severe mental illness;

- those who have had a severe stroke affecting both the arm and leg on one side or those who are paraplegic.

The new rules state that 'people receiving certain regular treatments are treated as incapable of work on any day on which they are engaged in that treatment'. Among the treatments mentioned by the rules is 'regular weekly treatment by way of haemodialysis or peritoneal dialysis for chronic renal failure'. Haemodialysis patients would therefore be regarded as incapable of work on two or three days a week, and can claim benefit for those days.

Income Support and Tax Credits

Those who are unemployed or off sick but have *not* paid National Insurance Contributions, may be able to get Income Support if the household income falls below the minimum set by DWP. Your needs are calculated according to your circumstances, such as number of children, degree of disability etc. So it is impossible to give an amount here. If you qualify for Income Support, you get extra money, plus other benefits such as payment of fares to hospital. You may also get Housing Benefit and Community Charge rebate.

If you have children or are working, even if part time, you may qualify for Child and/or Working Tax Credit. Many Pensioners qualify for Pension Tax Credit. See your local Welfare Rights Agency or Citizens Advice Bureau.

Disability Living Allowance (DLA)

Disability Living Allowance has two separate parts. You may qualify for one or the other or both.

The first is for help with '*personal care*' (that is, if you need help with washing, dressing, toileting or with health care, such as taking medication or performing dialysis). There are three rates for this:

- **The lowest rate** is for those who are unable to get themselves a home-prepared midday meal, but can manage other aspects of personal care.

- **The middle rate** is for those who need approximately 35 hours per week of attention from another person to attend to personal care needs, during the daytime.

- **The highest rate** is payable for people who not only need help during the day, but also need frequent attention to their personal care during the night.

The second part of the Disability Living Allowance is concerned with mobility. This is payable if you find it very hard to get around. There are two rates of the mobility component.

- The **lower rate** is payable to people who cannot leave the house on their own. This is often successfully claimed by those who are registered blind or partially sighted, or those who may become suddenly unconscious without warning, such as some sufferers from epilepsy or diabetes. Mental health problems, such as severe panic attacks or agoraphobia, may also enable someone to qualify.

- The **higher rate** is payable to those have severe physical problems with walking. This is defined as being 'unable or nearly unable to walk'.

It is worth applying for the higher rate if you can manage only 50 yards before needing a pause due to breathlessness, fatigue or pain. To qualify you must be 65 or under, but once you have qualified you get the allowance until the age of 80.

If you qualify for the higher rate, you will also be entitled to road tax exemption and a disabled sticker for parking. This is quite hard to obtain unless you get Mobility Allowance, and may entail a letter from your doctor.

Attendance Allowance
If you are over the age of 65, you cannot get Disability Living Allowance. However, if you have personal care needs, you can get Attendance Allowance, according to the same rules as the personal care rates for Disability Living Allowance. You cannot claim for any mobility needs.

Neither Disability Living Allowance nor Attendance Allowance are taxable or means tested.

Invalid Care Allowance
This is an allowance paid to somebody who cares for someone receiving Attendance or Disability Living Allowance at the middle or higher rate. You should not be working for more than 16 hours a week, and must be providing the care for at least 35 hours a week. It is possible to earn up to a certain level and still claim the allowance, but it is taxable, and will count against any Income Support you may receive.

Financial help from the hospital

Payment of fares
If you get Income Support or a Tax Credit, you can claim fares to hospital at the General Office. Bring receipts or tickets showing what you have had to pay, plus proof of entitlement (your Income Support or Family Tax

Credit book, or reference number). Unfortunately, they cannot pay the costs of visiting a relative in hospital, but a grant for this can sometimes be given by the local Social Security office. If this is not available, there may be a charitable fund provided by your local Kidney Patient Association.

Even if you do not qualify for Income Support or Family Tax Credit, some units arrange to pay petrol money for journeys to attend dialysis treatment if this is done at your own expense. Ask in your unit.

Hardship grants

Many kidney units have a Patients' Association, which may be able to make grants of money to help in emergencies. These are almost always one-off payments rather than a regular sum.

There are national kidney charities which also make grants for hardship, holidays and other needs. Most requests will be considered. The best known are the NKRF (National Kidney Research Fund) and the BKPA (British Kidney Patient Association). People who have had kidney transplants can contact the Transplant Association of Great Britain. For addresses and telephone numbers, see Appendix 3.

Appendix 2
Further reading

Dr Sarah Brewer,
   Intimate Relations: Living and loving in later life. Age Concern Books
Dr Stewart A Cameron,
   Kidney Failure: The facts. Oxford University Press
Eileen Inge Herzberg,
   Know Your Complementary Therapies. Age Concern Books
Hugh Marriott,
   The Selfish Pig's Guide to Caring. Polperro Heritage Press
National Kidney Federation (in association with Amgen),
   Food with Thought. Available from the NKF
Toni Smith and Nicky Thomas,
   Renal Nursing. Bailliere-Tindall
Professor Peter Sönksen, Professor Charles Fox and Sue Judd,
   Diabetes: the 'at your fingertips' guide. Class Publishing
Dr Andy Stein and Janet Wild,
   Kidney Dialysis and Transplants: the 'at your fingertips' guide.
   Class Publishing
Dr Andy Stein and Janet Wild,
   Kidney Kidney Failure Explained. Class Publishing, London

Appendix 3
Useful addresses

Action on Smoking and Health (ASH)
102 Clifton Street
London EC2A 4HW
Tel: 020 7739 5902
Fax: 020 7613 0531
Helpline: 0800 169 0169
Website: www.ash.org.uk
Provides information on how smoking affects medical conditions.

Age Concern
Astral House
1268 London Road
London SW16 4EW
Tel: 020 8679 8000
Fax: 020 8766 07211
Helpline: 0800 009 0966
Website: www.ace.org.uk
Researches into the needs of older people, and is involved in policy making. Publishes many books, has useful fact sheets on a wide range of issues from benefits to care, and provides services via local branches.

British Association for Counselling and Psychotherapy
1 Regent Place
Rugby
Warwickshire CV21 2PJ
Helpline: 0870 443 5252
Website: www.bacp.co.uk
Publishes a directory of counsellors and psychotherapists in the UK.

British Complementary Medicine Association (BCMA)
249 Fosse Road South
Leicester LE3 1AE
Tel: 0116 282 5511
Website: www.bcma.co.uk
Publishes BCMA National Practitioner Register listing practitioners who belong to member organisations.

British Holistic Medical Association (BHMA)
59 Lansdowne Place
Hove
East Sussex BN3 1FL
Tel: 01273 725951
Website: www.bhma-sec.dircon.co.uk
For directory of members and book/tape list.

British Kidney Patient Association (BKPA)
Bordon
Hampshire GU35 9JZ
Tel: 01420 472021
Fax: 01420 4735831
Website: www.bkpa.org.uk
Provides information and advice to people with kidney illnesses throughout the UK. Grants available.

Carers UK
20–25 Glasshouse Yard
London EC1A 4JS
Tel: 020 7490 8818
Fax: 020 7490 8824
CarersLine: 0808 808 7777
Website: www.carersonline.org.uk
Offers information and support to all
people who have to care for others due to
medical or other problems.

Carers Scotland
91 Mitchell Street
Glasgow G1 3LN
Tel: 0141 221 9141
Fax: 0141 221 914o
CarersLine: 0808 808 7777
Website: www.carersonline.org.uk
Offers information and support to all
people in Scotland who have to care for
others due to medical or other problems.

Crossroads Care
10 Regent Place
Rugby
Warwickshire CV21 2PN
Tel: 01788 573653
Fax: 01788 565498
Website: www.crossroads.org.uk
Supports and delivers high quality
services for carers and people with care
needs, via a network of local branches.

Cruse – Bereavement Care
126 Sheen Road
Richmond
Surrey TW9 1UR
Tel: 020 8940 4818
Fax: 020 8940 7638
Website: www.crusebereavementcare.org.uk
Offers information on bereavement, sells
literature and has local branches which
can provide one-to-one counselling.

**Department for Work
and Pensions (DWP)**
Room 540
The Adelphi
1–11 John Adam Street
London WC2N 6HT
Tel: 020 7712 2171
Fax: 020 7712 2386
Benefits Enquiry Line: 0800 88 22 00
Website: www.dfwp.gov.uk

Depression Alliance
35 Westminster Bridge Road
London SE1 7JB
Tel: 020 7928 9992
Fax: 020 7633 0557
Website: www.depressionalliance.org
Offers information, support and under-
standing to anyone affected by depression
and relatives who want help. Has a net-
work of self-help groups, correspondence
schemes and a range of literature.

Diabetes UK
10 Queen Anne Street
London W1G 9LH
Tel: 020 7323 1531
Fax: 020 7637 3644
Helpline: 020 7636 6112
Provides advice and information on
diabetes; has local support groups.

Disability Alliance
Universal House
88–94 Wentworth Street
London E1 7SA
Tel: 020 7247 8776
Fax: 020 7247 8765
Rights Advice Line
Tel: 020 2247 8763
Campaigns for the rights of people with a
disability, and provides information and
advice.

Disabled Living Centres Council
Redbank House
4 St Chads Street
Manchester M8 8QA
Tel: 0161 834 1044
Website: www.dlce.org.uk
For Disabled Living Centres nearest you,
where you can see aids and equipment.

Disabled Living Foundation
380–384 Harrow Road
London W9 2HU
Tel: 020 7289 6111
Fax: 020 7266 2922
Helpline: 0870 603 9177
Website: www.dlf.org.uk
Provides information on all kinds of
equipment for people with special needs.

Employment Opportunities
for People with Disabilities
123 Minories
London EC3N 1NT
Tel: 020 7841 2727
Fax: 020 7841 9797
Website: www.opportunities.org.uk

Eurodial
Website: www.eurodial.org
The international dialysis organisation
dedicated to the care and mobility of
dialysis patients in Europe.

Free Prescriptions Advice Line
Tel: 0800 9177 711
(Mon–Fri 8am–6pm;
Sat & Sun 10am–4pm)
Advice on entitlement to free
prescriptions, dental and optical care.

Globaldialysis
Website: www.globaldialysis.com
Gives details of holiday and travel
information for dialysis patients.

Help the Aged
16–18 St James's Walk
London EC1R 0BE
Tel: 020 7278 1114
Website: www.helptheaged.org.uk
Provides advice and support for older
people and for carers.

Holiday Care
Imperial Buildings, 2nd Floor
Horley
Surrey RH6 7PZ
Tel: 01293 774 535
Fax: 01293 784 647
Information and advice about holidays,
travel or respite care, for older or disabled
people and their carers.

Institute of Complementary Medicine
(ICM)
PO Box 194
London SE16 7QZ
Tel: 020 7237 5165
Advice and details of specialist
organisations.

Kidney Cancer UK
11 Hathaway Road
Tile Hill Village
Coventry CV4 9HW
Tel: 02476 470 584
Website: www.kcuk.org
Information and support for people with
kidney cancer and their carers. Chat
room available via the website.

Kidney Patient Information Websites
Website: www.kidneydirections.com
Information and kidney patients and suggestions for ways to plan treatment.

Website: www.kidneypatientguide.org.uk
Information for people with kidney failure and for those who care for them.

Website: www.kidneywise.com
Advice and support for people affected by kidney failure.

Macmillan Cancer Relief
89 Albert Embankment
London SE1 7UQ
Tel: 020 7840 7840
Fax: 020 7840 7841
Helpline: 0808 808 0000
Website: www.cancerlink.org
Helps cancer patients, carers and families with practical and emotional support.

Medic-Alert Foundation
1 Bridge Wharf
156 Caledonian Road
London N1 9UU
Tel: 020 7833 3034
Fax: 020 7213 5653
Helpline: 0808 808 0000
e-mail: info@medicalert.co.uk
Offers a selection of jewellery with internationally recognised medical symbol. Runs a 24-hour emergency phoneline.

MIND (National Association for Mental Health)
Granta House
15–19 Broadway
London E15 4BQ
Tel: 0845 766 0163 (Monday–Friday, 9.15am–4.45pm)
Website: www.mind.org.uk
Information service for all matters relating to mental health.

National College of Hypnosis and Psychotherapy
12 Cross Street
Nelson
Lancashire BB9 7EN
Tel: 01282 699378
Publishes an annual directory of practitioners.

National Kidney Federation
6 Stanley Street
Worksop
Nottinghamshire S81 7HX
Tel: 01909 487795
Fax: 01909 481723
Helpline: 0845 601 0209
Website: www.kidney.org.uk
e-mail: nkf@kidney.org.uk
Aims to promote, throughout the UK, the welfare of people suffering from kidney disease or renal failure, and those relatives or friends who care for them.

National Kidney Research Fund
King's Chambers
Priestgate
Peterborough PE1 1FG
Tel: 01733 704650
Fax: 01733 704692
Helpline: 0845 300 1499
Website: www.nkrf.org.uk
e-mail: enquiries@nkrf.org.uk
Funds research into kidney disease, its causes and treatment. Works to raise awareness of kidney disease.

NHS Direct
Tel: 0845 46 47
Website: www.nhsdirect.nhs.uk
A 24-hour nurse-led helpline providing confidential healthcare advice and information.

NHS Organ Donor Information Service
Tel: 0845 6060 400
Website: www.nhsorgandonor.net
Provides information about donating organs, and how patients can benefit from organ donation.

Patients' Association
PO Box 935
Harrow
Middlesex HA1 3YJ
Tel: 020 8423 9111
Fax: 020 8423 9119
Helpline: 0845 608 4455
Website: www.patients-association.com
Provides advice on patients' rights.

Quitline
Tel: 0800 002 200
A freephone helpline that provides confidential and practical advice for people wanting to give up smoking.

Relate
Herbert Gray College
Little Church Street
Rugby
Warwickshire CV21 3AP
Tel: 01788 573241
Fax: 01788 535007
Helpline: 09069 123 715
Website: www.relate.org.uk
Formerly the Marriage Guidance Council. Offers relationship counselling at most branches.

Relatives & Residents Association
5 Tavistock Place
London WC1H 9SN
Tel: 020 7916 6055
Website: www.relres.org.uk
Offers information, practical advice and a forum for discussion and engagement to people (and their relatives) entering long-term care.

Renal Registry of the United Kingdom
Southmead Hospital
Southmead Road
Bristol BS10 5NB
Tel: 0117 959 5665
Fax: 0117 959 5664
Website: www.renalreg.com
Collects, analyses and presents data about the incidence, clinical management and outcome of renal disease.

Sexual Dysfunction Association
Windmill Place Business Centre
2-4 Windmill Lane
Southall
Middlesex UB2 4HJ
Helpline: 0870 774 3571
Website: www.impotence.org.uk
Offers help and advice on sexual problems.

The Samaritans
46 Marshall Street
London W1V 1LR
Tel: 08457 90 90 90
Textphone: 08457 90 91 92
(24 hours every day)
Offers confidential emotional support to
any person who is suicidal or despairing.

UK Transplant
Communications Directorate
Fox Den Road
Stoke Gifford
Bristol BS34 8RR
Tel: 0117 975 7575
Fax: 0117 975 7577
Website: www.uktransplant.org.uk

United Kingdom Home Care
Association (UKHCA)
42B Banstead Road
Carshalton Beeches
Surrey SM5 3NW
Tel: 020 8288 1551
For information about organisations
providing home care in your area.

United Kingdom Register
of Counsellors
PO Box 1050
Rugby
Warwickshire CV21 2HZ
Tel: 0870 443 5232
Fax: 0870 443 5161
Part of the British Association for
Counselling and Psychotherapy
Regulatory Body which provides details
of registered counsellors who offer safe
and accountable practice.

Vehicle Excise Duty (Road Tax)
DLA Unit
Warbreck House
Warbreck Hill Road
Blackpool FY2 0YE
Tel: 08457 123456
Information about exemption from road
tax for vehicles used exclusively by or for
disabled people.

Winged Fellowship Trust
Angel House
20–32 Pentonville Road
London N1 9XD
Tel: 020 7833 2594
Website: www.wft.org.uk
Provides respite care and holidays for
physically disabled people, with or
without a partner.

Glossary

This glossary provides brief explanations of the various technical words used in this book. Words printed in **bold italic type** have their own glossary entry.

Abdomen The lower part of the trunk, below the chest. Commonly referred to as the tummy or belly.

Access A method of gaining entry to the bloodstream to allow **dialysis**. Access methods used for **haemodialysis** include a **catheter, fistula** or graft.

Alfacalcidol A **vitamin D** supplement.

Anaemia A shortage of red blood cells in the body, causing tiredness, shortness of breath and pale skin.

APD Abbreviation for automated peritoneal dialysis. A form of **peritoneal dialysis** that uses a machine to drain the dialysis fluid out of the patient and replace it with fresh solution. APD is usually carried out overnight while the patient is sleeping.

Arteries Blood vessels that carry blood from the heart to the rest of the body.

Artificial kidney Another name for the **dialyser** or filtering unit of a dialysis machine.

Biopsy A test involving the removal of a small piece of a kidney or other body tissue, so it can be examined under a microscope.

Bladder The organ in which urine is stored before being passed from the body.

Blood cells The microscopically tiny units that form the solid part of the blood. There are three main types: red blood cells, white blood cells and platelets.

Blood group An inherited characteristic of red blood cells. The common classification is based on whether or not a person has certain antigens (called A and B) on their cells. People belong to one of four blood groups, called A, B, AB and O.

Blood pressure The pressure that the blood exerts against the walls of the arteries as it flows through them. Blood pressure measurements consist of two numbers. The first shows the systolic blood pressure (as the heart beats), the second shows the diastolic blood pressure (between beats). One of the functions of the kidneys is to help control blood pressure.

Blood vessels The tubes that carry blood around the body. The main blood vessels are the **arteries** and **veins**.

Calcium A mineral that strengthens the bones. It is contained in some foods, including dairy products. It is stored in the bones and is present in the blood. The kidneys normally help to keep calcium in the bones. In kidney failure, calcium drains out of the bones, and the level of calcium in the blood falls.

CAPD Abbreviation for continuous ambulatory *peritoneal dialysis*. A continuous form of PD in which patients perform the exchanges of dialysis fluid by hand. The fluid is usually exchanged four times during the day, and is left inside the patient overnight.

Catheter A flexible plastic tube used to enter the interior of the body. A catheter is one of the access options for patients on *haemodialysis*. For patients on *peritoneal dialysis*, a catheter allows dialysis fluid to be put into and removed from the peritoneal cavity. A catheter may also be used to drain urine from the *bladder*.

Cholesterol A lipid (fat) that contributes towards damage of the *arteries*.

Ciclosporin An *immunosuppressant drug* used to prevent the *rejection* of a transplant kidney.

Creatinine A waste substance produced by the muscles when they are used. The name creatinine is also given to a blood test that measures the blood level of creatinine.

Diabetes A condition in which there is too much sugar in the blood. Whether this type of diabetes is controlled by insulin, tablets or diet, it can eventually cause kidney failure

Dialyser The filtering unit of a *dialysis machine*. It provides the dialysis membrane for patients on *haemodialysis*. The dialyser removes body wastes and excess water from the blood in a similar way to a normal kidney.

Dialysis An artificial process by which the toxic waste products of food and excess water are removed from the body. Dialysis therefore takes over some of the work normally performed by healthy kidneys.

Dialysis fluid The liquid that provides the 'container' into which toxic waste products and excess water pass during dialysis, for removal from the body.

Dialysis machine The machine used to perform haemodialysis. It includes a *dialyser*, which filters the patient's blood. The machine helps to pump the patient's blood through the dialyser, and monitors the dialysis process as it takes place.

Dialysis membrane A thin layer of tissue or plastic with many tiny holes in it, through which the process of dialysis takes place. In *peritoneal dialysis*, the patient's *peritoneum* provides the dialysis membrane. For *haemodialysis*, the dialysis membrane is made of synthetic material. In each case, the membrane keeps the dialysis fluid separate from the blood, while tiny holes in the membrane make it semi-permeable, allowing water and various substances to pass through it.

Diuretics Also referred to as water tablets, these drugs increase the amount of urine that is passed. Two commonly used diuretics are frusemide and bumetanide.

Donor A person who donates (gives) an organ to another person (the recipient).

Dry weight The weight of the body when it does not contain excess water in the tissues. Following *dialysis*, patients should return to their dry weight. If patients gain or lose 'flesh' weight, their dry weight needs to be recalculated to enable the correct amount of fluid to be removed during dialysis.

End-stage renal failure (ESRF) A term for advanced chronic kidney failure. People who develop ESRF will die within a few weeks unless treated by *dialysis* or a *transplant*.

Erythropoeitin (EPO) A hormone, made by the kidneys, which stimulates the bone marrow to produce red blood cells. In kidney failure, EPO is not made and *anaemia* results.

Fistula An enlarged vein, usually at the wrist or elbow, that gives *access* to the bloodstream for *haemodialysis*. The fistula is created by joining a vein to an artery in a small operation. This increases the flow of blood through the vein and causes it to enlarge, making it suitable for haemodialysis needles.

Fluid balance A state in which the body contains water and substances such as salts and minerals in the correct proportions. It is maintained by the efficient removal of waste products and water by healthy kidneys, or by a process (such as *dialysis*) that performs their job for them.

Glomerulonephritis Inflammation of the glomeruli, which is one of the causes of kidney failure.

Haemodialysis A form of dialysis in which the blood is cleaned outside the body, in a machine called a *dialysis machine* or kidney machine. Each dialysis session lasts 3–5 hours, and sessions are usually needed three times a week.

Haemodialysis unit The part of a hospital where patients go for haemodialysis.

Haemoglobin (Hb) A substance in red blood cells that carries oxygen around the body. Blood levels of haemoglobin are measured to look for *anaemia*. A low Hb level indicates anaemia.

Immune system The body's natural defence system. It includes organs (such as the spleen and appendix), lymph nodes (including the 'glands' in the neck) and specialist white blood cells called lymphocytes. The immune system protects the body from infections, foreign bodies and cancer.

Immunosuppressant drugs To prevent rejection of a transplant kidney, it is necessary for patients to take immunosuppressant drugs which dampen down the immune system. Commonly used examples are ciclosporin, azathioprine, prednisolone and (more recently) tacrolimus.

Kidney failure A condition in which the kidneys are less able than normal to perform their functions of removing toxic wastes, removing excess water, helping to control blood pressure, helping to control red blood cell manufacture and helping to keep the bones strong and healthy. Advanced chronic kidney failure is called *end-stage renal failure (ESRF)*.

Peritoneal cavity The area between the two layers of the peritoneum inside the *abdomen*. The peritoneal cavity contains the abdominal organs, including the stomach, liver and bowels. It normally contains only about 100 ml of liquid, but expands easily to provide a reservoir for *dialysis fluid* in *PD*.

Peritoneal dialysis (PD) A form of dialysis that takes place inside the patient's *peritoneal cavity*, using the *peritoneum* as the dialysis membrane. Bags of dialysis fluid are drained in and out of the peritoneal cavity via a PD catheter.

Peritoneum A natural membrane that lines the inside of the wall of the abdomen and that covers all the abdominal organs (the stomach, bowels, liver, etc.)

Peritonitis Inflammation of the *peritoneum*, caused by an infection. People on *PD* risk getting peritonitis if they touch the connection between their PD catheter and the bags of dialysis fluid. Most attacks are easily treated with antibiotic drugs.

Phosphate A mineral that helps *calcium* to strengthen the bones.

Polycystic kidney disease (PCKD) A disease that runs in families in which both kidneys are full of cysts (abnormal lumps). PCKD is one of the causes of kidney failure.

Potassium A mineral that is normally present in the blood. Either too much or too little potassium can be dangerous, causing the heart to stop. People with kidney failure may need to restrict the amount of potassium in their diet.

Rejection The process by which a patient's immune system recognises a transplant kidney (or other transplanted organ) as not its 'own', then tries to destroy it and remove it from the body.

Renal Adjective meaning relating to the kidneys.

Renal unit A hospital department that treats disorders of the kidneys.

Statin A drug to lower the level of *cholesterol* in the blood.

Tissue type A set of inherited characteristics on the surface of cells. Each person's tissue type has six components (three from each parent). Although there are only three main sorts of tissue type characteristic (called A, B and DR), each of these comes in 20 or more different versions. The more characteristics that match, the more likely is a transplant to succeed.

Transplant A term used to mean either a transplant kidney (or other organ) or a transplant operation.

Transplant waiting list A system, co-ordinated nationally, that seeks to find the 'right' transplant organ for the 'right' patient. The average waiting time for a transplant kidney is about two years.

Urea A substance made by the liver. It is one of the waste products from food that builds up in the blood when someone has kidney failure.

Veins Blood vessels which carry blood from the body back to the heart.

Vitamin D A chemical that helps the body to absorb calcium from the diet. Blood levels of vitamin D are usually low in people with kidney failure.

Index

The *Class Health* Feedback Form

We hope that you found this **Class Health** book helpful. We always appreciate readers' opinions and would be grateful if you could take a few minutes to complete this form for us.

1 How did you acquire your copy of this book?

From my local library ☐

Read an article in a newspaper/magazine ☐

Found it by chance ☐

Recommended by a friend ☐

Recommended by a patient organisation/charity ☐

Recommended by a doctor/nurse/advisor ☐

Saw an advertisement ☐

2 How much of the book have you read?

All of it ☐

More than half of it ☐

Less than half of it ☐

3 Which copies/chapters have been most helpful?

....

....

4 Overall, how useful to you was this *Class Health* book?

Extremely useful ☐

Very useful ☐

Useful ☐

5 What did you find most helpful?

....

....

6 What did you find least helpful?

....

....

7 **Have you read any other health books?**

Yes ☐   No ☐

If yes, which subjects did they cover?

....

....

....

How did this *Class Health* book compare?

Much better   ☐

Better   ☐

About the same   ☐

Not as good   ☐

8 **Would you recommend this book to a friend?**

Yes ☐   No ☐

Thank you for your help. Please send your completed form to:

Class Publishing, FREEPOST, London W6 7BR

Surname _____ First name _____

Title Prof/Dr/Mr/Mrs/Ms _____

Address _____

Town _____ Postcode _____ Country _____

☐ Please add my name and address to receive details of related books
[*Please note, we will not pass on your details to any other company*]

Have you found **Living Well with Kidney Failure** *useful and practical? If so, you may be interested in other books from Class Publishing.*

Kidney Failure Explained   £14.99

Dr Andy Stein and Janet Wild

The complete and updated reference manual for people suffering from kidney failure, which tells you everything you need to know about the condition. This is a book for anyone with kidney problems, their families and friends and those who look after the needs of people with a kidney condition, including GPs, practice nurses and specialist nurses.

> *'I believe this excellent book should be read by every kidney patient and their family. I can recommend it without hesitation.'*
> Austin Donohoe, Chairman,
> National Kidney Federation

Heart Health – the 'at your fingertips' guide   £14.99

Dr Graham Jackson

This practical handbook, written by a leading cardiologist, answers all your questions about heart conditions. It tells you all about you and your heart; how to keep your heart healthy, or if it has been affected by heart disease – how to make it as strong as possible.

> *'Those readers who want to know more about the various treatments for heart disease will be much enlightened.'*
> Dr James Le Fanu, *Daily Telegraph*

Sexual Health for Men – the 'at your fingertips' guide   £14.99

Dr Philip Kell and Vanessa Griffiths

This practical handbook answers hundreds of real questions from men with erectile dysfunction and their partners. Up to 50% of the population aged over 60 is impotent – though they need not be, if they take appropriate action.

Kidney Dialysis and Transplants – the 'at your fingertips' guide   £14.99

Dr Andy Stein and Janet Wild with Juliet Auer

A practical handbook for anyone (and the families of those) with long-term kidney failure. The book contains answers to over 450 real questions actually asked by people with end-stage renal failure, and offers positive, clear and medically accurate advice on every aspect of living with the condition.

> *'A first class book on kidney dialysis and transplants that is simple and accurate, and can be used to equal advantage by doctors and their patients.'*
> Dr Thomas Stuttaford, *The Times*

High Blood Pressure – the 'at your fingertips' guide   £14.99

Dr Tom Fahey, Professor Deirdre Murphy with Dr Julian Tudor Hart

The authors use all their years of experience as blood pressure experts to answer your questions on high blood pressure, in order to give you the information you need to bring your blood pressure down – and keep it down.

> *'Readable and comprehensive information'*
> Dr Sylvia McLaughlan, Director
> General, The Stroke Association

Beating Depression – the 'at your fingertips' guide   £17.99

Dr Stefan Cembrowicz and Dr Dorcas Kingham

Depression is one of most common illnesses in the world – affecting up to one in four people at some time in their lives. Beating Depression shows sufferers and their families that they are not alone, and offers tried and tested techniques for overcoming depression.

PRIORITY ORDER FORM

Cut out or photocopy this form and send it (post free in the UK) to:

Class Publishing Priority Service
FREEPOST
London W6 7BR

Please send me urgently (*tick boxes below*)	*Post included* *price per copy (UK only)*

☐ **Living Well with Kidney Failure** £17.99
(ISBN 1 85959 112 4)

☐ **Kidney Failure Explained** £17.99
(ISBN 1 85959 070 5)

☐ **Kidney Dialysis and Transplants – the 'at your fingertips' guide** £17.99
(ISBN 1 85959 046 2)

☐ **Heart Health – the 'at your fingertips' guide** £17.99
(ISBN 1 85959 097 7)

☐ **High Blood Pressure – the 'at your fingertips' guide** £17.99
(ISBN 1 85959 090 X)

☐ **Sexual Health for Men – the 'at your fingertips' guide** £17.99
(ISBN 1 85959 011 X)

☐ **Beating Depression – the 'at your fingertips' guide** £20.99
(ISBN 1 85959 063 2)

TOTAL _____

Easy ways to pay

Cheque: I enclose a cheque payable to Class Publishing for £ _____

Credit card: Please debit my ☐ Mastercard ☐ Visa ☐ Amex

Number _____ Expiry date _____

Name _____

My address for delivery is _____

_____

Town _____ County _____ Postcode _____

Telephone number (*in case of query*) _____

Credit card billing address if different from above _____

_____

Town _____ County _____ Postcode _____

Class Publishing's guarantee: remember that if, for any reason, you are not satisfied with these books, we will refund all your money, without any questions asked. Prices and VAT rates may be altered for reasons beyond our control.